National Diet and Nutrition Survey:

children aged 1½ to 4½ years

Volume 2: Report of the dental survey

A survey carried out in Great Britain on behalf of the Departments of Health by the Social Survey Division of the Office of Population Censuses and Surveys

Kerstin Hinds

Janet R Gregory

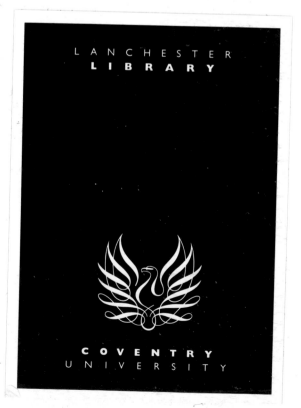

London: HMSO

© *Crown copyright 1995*
First published 1995

ISBN 0 11 691612 5

Printed in the United Kingdom for HMSO
Dd 0300400   C18   3/95   65536   3400   317775   10/32357

Foreword

I very much welcome this dental report which is the first, in many years, to survey extensively the dental health of pre-school children aged $1^{1}/_{2}$ to $4^{1}/_{2}$ years.

The report has an important place in the programme of National Diet and Nutrition Surveys and I am pleased that the opportunity has been taken to use the same age sample to look at oral health. It is at this age, when primary teeth are becoming fully functional, that good eating habits should be established.

The information gathered will be particularly useful in planning the future delivery of oral health care and take forward the objectives and initiatives set out in national and local oral health strategies.

Gerald Malone
Minister for Health
Department of Health

Contents

Page

Foreword iii

Acknowledgements vii

Notes viii

Summary of main findings ix

1 Background and research design 1
1.1 Background to the survey 1
1.2 The purpose and design of the dental survey 1
1.3 The sample 1
1.4 The survey package 2
    1.4.1 The dental survey within the context of the NDNS 2
    1.4.2 The conduct of the dental survey 2
    1.4.3 The dental examination 2
    1.4.4 The dental interview 3
1.5 The response 3
1.6 Plan of the Report 3

2 Sample design, response and characteristics of respondents 5
2.1 Introduction 5
2.2 The dietary survey sample 5
2.3 Response to the dietary sift 5
2.4 Response to the dental survey in relation to response to the dietary survey 5
2.5 Response to elements of the dental survey 6
2.6 Response to elements of the survey by age and sex 7
2.7 Main characteristics of the dental survey sample compared with the dietary survey
    sample and the general population 7
    2.7.1 Social class 8
    2.7.2 Region 8
2.8 Other characteristics of the dental sample 8
    2.8.1 Mother's highest educational qualification 9
    2.8.2 Family type 9
    2.8.3 Working mothers and child-care arrangements 10
    2.8.4 Employment status of head of household 10
    2.8.5 Receipt of benefits 10
2.9 Conclusion 10

3 Condition of young children's teeth 11
3.1 Introduction 11
3.2 Prevalence of dental decay 11
    3.2.1 The proportion of children with active decay, filled teeth, teeth
    missing due to decay and with any decay experience 11
    3.2.2 Variations in dental decay by characteristics of children and their households 11
    3.2.3 Decay into the dental pulp 14
3.3 The number of teeth with decay experience 14
    3.3.1 The mean number of teeth with decay experience for all children 14
    3.3.2 The mean number of teeth with experience of decay for children with some
    decayed teeth 16
    3.3.3 The range in the number of teeth with decay experience 17
    3.3.4 Decay into the dental pulp 17
3.4 Decay on molars, incisors and canines 17
3.5 Treatment of decay 18
3.6 Distribution of tooth conditions around the mouth 18

4 Dental care and advice 21
4.1 Introduction 21
4.2 Visits to dentist 21
4.3 Advice received by parents on dental care issues 21
    4.3.1 Type of advice 22
    4.3.2 Source of advice 23
4.4 Teething 23
    4.4.1 Degree of difficulty teething 23
    4.4.2 Use of teething aids 23
4.5 Toothbrushing 24
4.6 Fluoride use 27
    4.6.1 Fluoride concentration of toothpaste used 27
    4.6.2 Amount of toothpaste used 28
    4.6.3 Use of fluoride supplements 29
    4.6.4 Use of fluoride supplements and fluoride advice 30
4.7 Mother's dental attendance pattern and child's visits to a dentist 30

5 The use of bottles, dinky feeders and dummies and the consumption of foods and drinks containing sugars 31
5.1 Introduction 31
5.2 The use of bottles 31
5.3 The use of dinky feeders 32
5.4 The use of dummies 33
5.5 Drinks in bed and during the night 33
5.6 Eating at night 35
5.7 Consumption of foods containing sugars 35
    5.7.1 Data from the dietary interview (food frequency questions) 35
    5.7.2 Data from the four-day weighed intake diary 35
5.8 Household expenditure on sweets and chocolates 38

6 Variations in patterns of decay 40
    Summary of chapter 40
6.1 Introduction 41
6.2 Measures associated with dental care and dental condition 41
    6.2.1 Toothbrushing 41
    6.2.2 Visits to the dentist 41
    6.2.3 Advice received by parents about caring for their child's teeth 42
    6.2.4 Use of fluoride supplements 42
    6.2.5 Mother's dental attendance pattern 43
6.3 Measures associated with eating and drinking and dental condition 43
    6.3.1 The use of bottles, dinky feeders and dummies 43
    6.3.2 Night-time drinking and eating practices at the time of interview 44
    6.3.3 Household spending on confectionery 44
    6.3.4 Dietary measures and dental condition 44
6.4 Independent relationships between behavioural variables and dental decay 49
    6.4.1 Dental care and dental decay 49
    6.4.2 Dietary behaviour and dental decay 49
6.5 Independent relationships between background characteristics of children and their households, dental behaviour and dental decay 49
6.6 Relationships between dietary behaviour and dental habits and decay experience 51

7 Trauma to the incisors and erosion of the upper incisors 52
7.1 Introduction 52
7.2 Trauma to the incisors 52
7.3 Erosion of the upper incisors 52

Appendices

A	*Dentist's criteria for the dental examination*	56
B	*Fieldwork documents*	58
C	*Tables associated with Chapter 5: Data on past use of bottles*	111
D	*Tables associated with Chapter 6: The mean number of teeth with experience of decay in relation to various dental care and dietary behaviour variables*	112
E	*Tables associated with Chapter 7: The proportion of children with erosion in relation to various background and behavioural characteristics*	115
F	*Sampling errors*	121
G	*Glossary of abbreviations, terms and survey definitions*	128
H	*Summary of the National Diet and Nutrition Survey of children aged 1 $^1/_2$ to 4 $^1/_2$ years Volume 1: Report of the Diet and Nutrition Survey*	132

List of tables and figures   140

Acknowledgements

We would like to thank everybody who contributed to the survey and the production of this report. We were supported by our specialist colleagues in OPCS who carried out the sampling, fieldwork, coding and editing stages.

Great thanks are due to the interviewers who worked on the survey and who showed such enthusiasm for the subject matter, and to the dentists who joined the interviewers to carry out the dental examinations.

Thanks go also to the following people who provided great assistance and specialist advice at various stages of the survey:

- Daniel Kelly, the main OPCS researcher during the initial stages of the survey

- Ian Cooper and Colin Howard from the Dental Division of the Department of Health in England

- Professor R J Anderson and Gillian Bradnock at the University of Birmingham Unit of Dental Public Health who advised on the dental examination and Dr J Nunn of the University of Newcastle-upon-Tyne Dental School for help with the training materials

- Dr P Clarke from the Nutrition Unit at the Department of Health

Most importantly, we would like to thank all the participants in the survey, both children and parents, who gave up so much of their time, made interviewers and dentists very welcome in their homes and showed a great deal of interest in the survey.

Notes

Tables showing percentages

In general, percentages are shown if the base is 30 or more. Where a base number is less than 30, actual numbers are shown within square brackets.

The row or column percentages may add to 99% or 101% because of rounding.

The varying positions of the percentage signs and bases in the tables denote the presentation of different types of information. Where there is a percentage sign at the head of a column and the base at the foot, the whole distribution is presented and the individual percentages add to between 99% and 101%. Where there is no percentage sign in the table and a note above the figures, the figures refer to the proportion of children who had the attribute being discussed, and the complimentary proportion, to add to 100%, is not shown in the table.

Where missing answers represented less than 1% of a distribution the percentages were recalculated on the base excluding missing cases, but the base including missing cases is presented for consistency. Where missing answers represented more than 1% of a distribution, 'don't know' or 'unclassified' are included as categories in the tables.

Conventions

The following conventions have been used within tables:
-   no cases
0   values less than 0.5%
[ ]   the numbers inside the square brackets are the actual number of observations when the total number of cases, that is the base, is fewer than 30.

Tables showing descriptive statistics - mean, percentiles, standard error of the mean, standard deviation

These are shown in tables to an appropriate number of decimal places.

Significant differences

Differences commented on the text are shown as being significant at the 99% or 95% confidence levels ($p<0.01$ and $p<0.05$). Throughout the Report the terms 'significant' and 'statistically significant' are used interchangeably. Where differences are described as being 'not statistically significant' this indicates that $p>0.05$. The formulae used to test for significant differences between percentages and means are shown in Appendix F.

Age groupings

For most analysis in this Report, children are grouped into three age groups; $1^1/_2$ to $2^1/_2$, $2^1/_2$ to $3^1/_2$ and $3^1/_2$ to $4^1/_2$ years. The precise definition of these groups is as follows:

$1^1/_2$ to $2^1/_2$ years	Less than 30 months at the time of the dental examination
$2^1/_2$ to $3^1/_2$ years	30 to 41 months inclusive at dental examination
$3^1/_2$ to $4^1/_2$ years	42 months and over at dental examination

A few children in the oldest age group were aged over $4^1/_2$ years at the time of the dental examination; the explanation for this is found in Chapter 1, section 1.3.

Summary of main findings

Introduction

This dental survey is the first in many years to investigate the dental health of a nationally representative sample of British preschool children. It was carried out as the final component of the National Diet and Nutrition Survey (NDNS) of children aged $1^1/_2$ to $4^1/_2$ years.[1]

The dental survey comprised a dental examination by a dentist seconded from the Community Dental Services of the National Health Service, and a dental interview. The examination included assessments for caries, trauma, or accidental damage, to the incisors and erosion of the upper incisors. The interview collected information on a range of topics including visits to the dentist, teething experiences, toothbrushing habits and the use of bottles, dinky feeders and dummies. Data relating to social and economic characteristics of children and their households were collected by questionnaire interview on the diet and nutrition survey and linked to the dental data. Some diet and nutrition survey data about dietary habits have also been linked to the dental data enabling investigation of a wide range of possible relationships between dietary behaviour and dental health (**Chapter 1**).

The sample for the diet and nutrition survey and hence the dental survey was selected using a multi-stage random probability design. A total of 1658 children participated in the dental survey, representing 89% of those who took part in the diet and nutrition survey and 79% of those originally selected as eligible for the diet and nutrition survey (the eligible sample). For some children consent was given to the dental interview but not to the examination and for some children partial rather than complete examinations were carried out. A total of 1532 children had a complete examination for the caries component of the dental examination, 73% of the eligible sample (**Chapter 2**).

Comparison of the characteristics of the responding sample with those of the total population and other large surveys showed very good agreement, confirming that the sample was representative of the population of children aged $1^1/_2$ to $4^1/_2$ years in private households in Britain. (**Chapter 2**).

Dental decay among children aged $1^1/_2$ to $4^1/_2$ years (Chapter 3)

Overall 17% of $1^1/_2$ to $4^1/_2$ year olds had some experience of dental decay. The proportion of children affected increased with age; 4% of $1^1/_2$ to $2^1/_2$ year olds, 14% of $2^1/_2$ to $3^1/_2$ year olds and 30% of those aged $3^1/_2$ to $4^1/_2$ years had some experience of dental decay. There was no variation in decay experience by sex. Most of children's decay experience was untreated or active decay. Only 2% of $1^1/_2$ to $4^1/_2$ year olds had filled teeth and 2% had teeth missing due to decay.

Overall children aged $1^1/_2$ to $2^1/_2$ years had an average of 0.1 teeth with decay experience, those aged $2^1/_2$ to $3^1/_2$ years had 0.5 teeth affected and an average of 1.3 teeth showed decay experience among those in the oldest age cohort.

A higher proportion of children in households where the head was in a manual social class group, as defined by occupation, had experience of dental decay than was found among those from non-manual backgrounds. Decay experience was also related to the highest educational qualifications of children's mothers with those whose mothers had no educational qualifications having highest experience of dental decay and those whose mothers had GCE 'A' levels or above having lowest decay experience.

Decay experience varied notably among children from different parts of Britain; Scottish children and those in the North of England had more decay than those in other parts of England and Wales. Half of the $3^1/_2$ to $4^1/_2$ year olds in Scotland and 43% of those in the Northern region of England had some experience of dental decay compared with less than a quarter of those in the rest of England and Wales.

Children living in lone-parent families, in households where the head was unemployed or economically inactive and in households where at least one adult was receiving Income Support or Family Credit were significantly more likely to have each type of dental decay than other children.

Dental care and advice (Chapter 4)

Prior to the survey, a quarter of $1^1/_2$ to $2^1/_2$ year olds, half the children aged $2^1/_2$ to $3^1/_2$ years and three quarters of those aged $3^1/_2$ to $4^1/_2$ years had been examined by a dentist.

Parents were asked whether they had received advice about what their child should be eating and drinking to look after their teeth, about cleaning their child's teeth and about giving or not giving their child fluoride drops or tablets; 60% had received advice on at least one of these issues and dentists and dental ancillaries were the main source of advice. Parents of children in Scotland were far more likely than those in other parts of Great Britain to have been advised to give their child fluoride drops or tablets; 65% of Scottish parents had received this advice compared with 24% of those in London and the South East, 18% in the Northern region and 12% in the Central and South West regions of England and Wales.

At the time of interview 98% of $1^1/_2$ to $4^1/_2$ year olds had started having their teeth brushed, either by an adult or themselves. For half the children in the survey toothbrushing started before the age of one year.

Most children sometimes brushed their own teeth and sometimes had their teeth brushed by an adult, however 10% of children had always brushed their own teeth. Over half the children in the survey (55%) had their teeth brushed (by self or other) more than once a day and one third had their teeth brushed once a day; 12% had their teeth brushed less than once a day.

Almost all children in the survey used fluoride toothpaste; about a third of children used toothpastes with low fluoride concentrations (below 600 parts per million). Eighteen per cent of children had used fluoride drops or tablets. The use of fluoride drops or tablets was more widespread in Scotland (over 50%) than elsewhere (less than 25%).

For many aspects of dental care, habits varied significantly for children with different social class backgrounds. Children from households with a non-manual head tended to have started toothbrushing at a younger age than those from manual backgrounds and they also brushed their teeth more frequently and were more likely to have been examined by a dentist prior to the survey.

The use of bottles, dinky feeders and dummies and the consumption of foods and drinks containing sugars (Chapter 5)

Overall 87% of children had used bottles at some time; 49% of those aged $1^1/_2$ to $2^1/_2$ years and 8% of those aged $3^1/_2$ to $4^1/_2$ years were reported to be current bottle users. Thirty one per cent of $1^1/_2$ to $2^1/_2$ year olds were using bottles every night as were 6% of those in the oldest age cohort. Over half the children using bottles at night usually had milk in them (56%) while a quarter (24%) usually had a drink containing non-milk extrinsic sugars including squashes, carbonated drinks and flavoured milks. [2]

Eighteen per cent of children had ever used a dinky feeder[3] and only 2% were said to be current users. Dinky feeders were mainly used during the day and drinks containing non-milk extrinsic sugars were most commonly consumed from them.

Just over half the children in the survey (53%) had ever used a dummy; only 5% of children had ever had a sweetened dummy.

The use of bottles, dinky feeders and dummies was more widespread among children from manual than from non-manual backgrounds.

At the time of the survey, just under a third of children (31%) were reported to have a drink in bed every night and almost half (48%) sometimes had a drink in bed. When drinking in bed, 12% of children usually had a drink containing non-milk extrinsic sugars; two thirds of these children had a drink every night.

Five per cent of children were reported ever to have something to eat in bed or during the night.

Overall 43% of children had sugar confectionery and 24% had carbonated drinks on at least most days of the week, at the time of the survey (data from the dietary survey interview); for both the proportions consuming with this frequency increased with age. Children from manual backgrounds were much more likely to be frequent consumers of sugar confectionery and carbonated drinks than were those from non-manual households.

Dental care, dietary behaviour and dental decay (Chapter 6)

The younger children were when they started having their teeth brushed or brushing their own teeth and the more frequently the teeth were brushed, the lower the proportion having tooth decay. For example, 12% of those whose teeth were brushed (by self or other) before the age of one year had experience of caries compared with 34% of those who did not start toothbrushing until after the age of 2 years. Decay prevalence was higher among children who always brushed their own teeth than among those where an adult sometimes or always brushed their teeth for them.

Children who had never used a bottle, dinky feeder or dummy had considerably less experience of dental decay than those who had (13% compared with 32%).

A higher proportion of those aged $1^1/_2$ to $2^1/_2$ and $2^1/_2$ to $3^1/_2$ years who had a drink in bed every night had decay experience than of those who had a drink in bed only sometimes or never. Among all children who consumed drinks in bed every night, 29% of those who had a drink containing non-milk extrinsic sugars had experience of decay compared with 11% of those who had milk.

For children of all ages the frequency of consumption of sugar confectionery and of carbonated drinks reported in the dietary interview at the time of the survey was related to dental decay; for example, 40% of $3^1/_2$ to $4^1/_2$ year olds who had sugar confectionery most days or more often had experience of caries compared with 22% of those who consumed sugar confectionery less frequently.

Trauma to the incisors and erosion of the upper incisors (Chapter 7)

The incisors of 15% of children aged $1^1/_2$ to $4^1/_2$ years had experienced trauma (accidental damage); there was little variation by age or sex. Most of the trauma affected teeth on the upper jaw, only 2% of children had experienced trauma to the lower incisors. Fractures were the most common type of trauma recorded; 59% of children with some dental trauma had a tooth which was fractured only as far as the enamel while 14% and 2% had teeth which were fractured into the dentine and dental pulp respectively. Eight per cent of children with some experience of trauma had lost a tooth through accidental damage.

Dental erosion has been defined as the loss of dental hard tissue by a chemical process that does not involve bacteria [4]. The main causes of dental erosion are thought to be dietary habits such as the consumption of demineralizing acidic foods. An attempt to assess the national prevalence of erosion has been undertaken only once before this survey; on the 1993 survey of children's dental health in the United Kingdom[5]. This survey used the same methodology as the 1993 children's dental health survey to investigate erosion. The upper incisors were examined on both the buccal (front) and palatal (back) surfaces and for each surface an assessment was made as to whether there was erosion into the enamel, erosion into the dentine or erosion into the dental pulp. Erosion, especially into the enamel only, can be difficult to identify and different dentists may have made different assessments.[6]

Erosion into the dentine or pulp affected the buccal surfaces of the teeth of 2% of children and the palatal surfaces of 8%. The prevalence of erosion increased with age, with 3% of children aged $1^1/_2$ to $2^1/_2$ years found to have some palatal erosion into the dentine or pulp compared with 13% of those aged $3^1/_2$ to $4^1/_2$ years.

For neither trauma nor erosion were differences identified by social class. Erosion was not found to be significantly related to dental care or dietary behaviour.

References and notes

[1] This survey of the diet and nutrition of British children aged $1^1/_2$ to $4^1/_2$ years forms part of the National Diet and Nutrition Survey programme, which was set up jointly by the Ministry of Agriculture, Fisheries and Food and the Department of Health to assess the dietary practices and nutritional status of different age groups within the British population. The dental component of this survey was commissioned from OPCS by the Department of Health. It is intended that dental surveys will also be linked to further surveys in the NDNS programme; these will focus on people aged 65 years and over, school children aged 5 to 15 years and adults aged 16 to 64 years. For information on the diets of preschool children see :
Gregory J R Collins D L Davies P S W Hughes J M Clarke P C. *National Diet and Nutrition Survey: children aged $1^1/_2$ to $4^1/_2$ years. Volume 1: Report of the diet and nutrition survey* HMSO (1995).

[2] Drinks containing non-milk extrinsic sugars included: fruit squash with sugar, blackcurrant drink (not diet), fruit juice or syrup, carbonated drinks (including low calorie carbonated drinks), hot chocolate, Ovaltine, Horlicks, flavoured milk, tea and coffee with sugar. A definition of non-milk extrinsic sugars is given in Appendix G.

[3] The term *dinky feeder* used in this report refers to the small comforter a child can be given, with a reservoir for small quantities of liquid behind the teat.

[4] Pindborg J J (1970) *Pathology of Dental Hard Tissues* Copenhagen: Munksgaarrd, pp 312-321.

[5] O'Brien M. *Children's Dental Health in the United Kingdom 1993* HMSO (1994).

[6] Further discussion of the methodology for the erosion examination is found in Chapter 7 of this Report and Appendix F of the report of the 1993 survey of schoolchildren's dental health.[5]

1 Background and research design

1.1 Background to the survey

This dental health survey of children aged $1\frac{1}{2}$ to $4\frac{1}{2}$ years is the first national survey of the dental condition of children of this age group (hereafter referred to as preschool children) since 1968 [1]. It has been carried out as one component of a much wider study, the 1992/93 *National Diet and Nutrition Survey (NDNS) of children aged $1\frac{1}{2}$ to $4\frac{1}{2}$ years*. This survey of more than 1500 preschool children living in England, Wales and Scotland, is part of a programme developed by the Ministry of Agriculture, Fisheries and Food and the Department of Health, to monitor the diets and nutritional status of representative samples of the population. The dental survey, commissioned by the Department of Health, used the same sample of children who took part in the diet and nutrition survey. [2] It was carried out among those whose parents, at the end of the dietary survey, consented to a request to a dental recall.

The Social Survey Division (SSD) of the Office of Population Censuses and Surveys (OPCS) carried out both the dietary and dental components of the National Diet and Nutrition Survey of children aged $1\frac{1}{2}$ to $4\frac{1}{2}$ years. The dental survey was designed in collaboration with the Unit of Dental Public Health at the University of Birmingham. SSD has considerable experience in undertaking national dental surveys including the recent survey, *Children's dental health in the United Kingdom, 1993*, [3] which investigated the dental condition of school children aged between 5 and 15 years, two previous children's dental health surveys conducted in 1973[4] and 1983[5] and the United Kingdom survey of adult dental health in 1988[6] which provided information on the dental condition of those aged 16 to 64 years, which could be compared with similar studies undertaken in the 1960s and 1970s.[7,8,9]

The National Diet and Nutrition Survey offered an excellent opportunity to produce a unique set of dental data for children aged $1\frac{1}{2}$ to $4\frac{1}{2}$ years; the information collected can stand alone, and be combined with the dietary information, thereby allowing a wide range of possible links between diet and tooth condition to be examined. Using the same sample of children for the dietary and dental surveys also had practical and cost advantages. In the NDNS programme, the survey of children aged $1\frac{1}{2}$ to $4\frac{1}{2}$ years will be followed by surveys of the diets of people aged 65 years and over, children aged 5 to 15 years, and adults aged 16 to 64 years; it is intended that oral health surveys will also be linked to these studies.

1.2 The purpose and design of the dental survey

The dental survey of children aged $1\frac{1}{2}$ to $4\frac{1}{2}$ years had five main aims:

1. To collect baseline information about the condition of preschool children's teeth, by examination

In this dental survey of preschool children, the main aim was to describe the condition of the teeth of children aged $1\frac{1}{2}$ to $4\frac{1}{2}$ years. This information may be used in setting targets for policy recommendations, and as baseline data against which to measure future changes in the dental health of preschool children. A dental examination was therefore central to the survey.

2. To investigate dental behaviour through an interview

The Department of Health is keen to identify common behaviour which might damage the teeth of children aged $1\frac{1}{2}$ to $4\frac{1}{2}$ years. In addition to the data from the examination, short interviews with the children's mothers or main carers were conducted to collect information on the drinks consumed and drinking vessels used by preschool children and on their consumption of sugars and dental cleaning practices. Comparing the condition of preschool children's teeth with their dental behaviour may provide information which could be used in formulating policies for dental care.

3. To enable future monitoring of the sample

As well as providing the data presented in this Report, the survey will enable the future dental health of this group of children to be monitored. This will be possible without further examinations in a survey context, by linking the survey data with treatment records held at Dental Practice Boards for all patients registered with dentists working in the General Dental Services of the National Health Service (NHS).[10] After the dental examination and interview, parents were asked to give written consent for their child's records to be flagged on the relevant Dental Practice Board's database to allow monitoring of all NHS dental treatment each child may undergo until the age of 16 years. In the future, analysis of this information might show how dental problems in young children progress through childhood, providing indicators that could be used to identify which preschool children are at greatest risk of future dental problems.

4. To investigate the prevalence of trauma and erosion in the deciduous incisors

Although the examination focused primarily on the prevalence of dental caries among the children examined, evidence of 'trauma' or accidental damage to teeth, and 'erosion' were also recorded during the examination.

5. To enable dental status to be correlated with dietary data

1.3 The sample

The preschool children included in the dental survey were sampled originally for the diet and nutrition survey. Eligible children were those aged $1\frac{1}{2}$ to $4\frac{1}{2}$ years at the mid-point of the fieldwork period, living in private, that is non-institutional, households in Great Britain.[11] The sample was designed so that each of the three age groups, $1\frac{1}{2}$ to $2\frac{1}{2}$, $2\frac{1}{2}$ to $3\frac{1}{2}$, $3\frac{1}{2}$ to $4\frac{1}{2}$ years, would contain enough children to allow separate analysis, by sex, with data being collected for about 1500 children in total. Only one eligible child was selected from any household to reduce the burden of participating in the survey on respondents and reduce the clustering of the data collected, so improving its accuracy.

A multi-stage random probability design was used to select the sample, with postal sectors as first stage units. The small users' Postcode Address File (PAF) was used as the sampling frame. This frame was stratified by region and by two variables from the 1981 census;[12] the proportion of heads of household in different socio-economic groups and the proportion of economically active females over the age of 16 years in private households.

One hundred sectors were selected as first stage units, with probability proportional to the number of postal delivery points. Forms were then sent to 280 randomly selected addresses in each sector, requesting details of the sex and date of birth of every person living at the address. From the returns, households containing an eligible child were identified. All eligible children identified by this process were included in the dietary survey, except where there was more than one eligible child in a household; in these cases, one child was selected at random before an interviewer visited the household.

Chapter 2 of this Report and Appendix C of the report of the preschool children's diet and nutrition survey[2] give more detailed information on the sample design.

1.4 The survey package

This section describes the dental survey within the context of the dietary survey package and then discusses the major organisational aspects of the dental survey. The components of the dental examination and the procedures used for examining preschool children are explained and the dental health topics included in the interview are summarised. Further details about the design of the NDNS may be found in Chapters 1 and 2 of the report of the diet and nutrition survey.[2]

1.4.1 The dental survey within the context of the NDNS

For ease of data collection, the dietary and dental components of the National Diet and Nutrition Survey were organised and conducted separately.

The dietary survey covered the following elements:
- a questionnaire interview to collect socio-economic and other background information
- a four-day weighed intake dietary record
- anthropometric measurements
- blood sample.

When the dietary survey was complete, interviewers asked if they could call on respondents again to carry out the dental survey. This comprised:
- a dental examination
- a dental questionnaire interview
- consent to monitoring future NHS dental treatment.

While a high degree of co-operation with all the different elements of the survey was important, the package was designed with a flexible structure that encouraged respondents to participate in as many elements as possible, but allowed for some aspects to be refused. For example, some parents and their children were willing to co-operate with all elements of the survey except the blood sample.

At the initial contact with the household, interviewers conducted the dietary questionnaire interview. Respondents were then asked to complete the four-day weighed intake record, weighing all the food and drink their child consumed both in and out of the home and recording this information, in great detail, in a diary. Those who participated in the dietary survey were only told about the dental component of the survey after all the elements of the dietary survey were complete to avoid any effect on response to the dietary components or on the quality of the dietary data being collected.

1.4.2 The conduct of the dental survey

When consent was given to the dental recall, the interviewer made an appointment to visit the child's home, accompanied by a dentist.

To avoid the possibility that the presence of a dentist might influence responses, dentists were asked to carry out the examination and then leave the home while the interviewer conducted the dental interview. When the examination and interview were complete, the interviewer sought written consent for the child's future NHS dental treatment to be monitored.

The main fieldwork for the dietary survey was carried out over a 12 month period from July 1992 to June 1993 to allow for possible seasonality of eating behaviour. Fieldwork was organised into four waves, each lasting about three months. So that the dietary data and dental data would relate to the same period, losses due to people moving would be minimised, and interviewers' rapport with children and families would be maintained, the dental data were collected shortly after the dietary data, in the last two weeks of each wave.

1.4.3 The dental examination

The examination covered three aspects of dental health of interest to the Department of Health. The dentists first identified which teeth were present in the mouth and examined them for caries. They then looked for evidence of trauma to the upper and lower incisors. Finally they examined the buccal and palatal surfaces of the upper incisors for erosion. Interviewers acted as recorders for the dentists.

The dentists who worked on the survey were recruited from the Community Dental Services of the NHS and all had experience of working with young children. Seventy nine dentists carried out survey examinations and it was important for them to use the same criteria when assessing the condition of children's teeth. Dental epidemiologists from the Universities of Birmingham and Newcastle-upon-Tyne developed written instructions for the dentists and assisted at one day briefings attended by interviewers and dentists, where the examination criteria were explained in more detail. Appendix A shows a copy of these criteria. The briefings did not provide an opportunity for dentists to examine preschool children, but they were shown slides of various conditions and told how to code marginal cases where opinions may have diverged. The interviewers attended the briefings to be trained in the procedure for charting (recording the examination codes on charts). The briefings took place shortly before the start of each wave of the dental survey and every dentist and interviewer attended at least one briefing. Refresher briefings were arranged for dentists who worked on more than one non-consecutive wave.

With a reasonably co-operative child, the examination was expected to last no longer than five minutes. Although protocol guidelines were given, dentists were free to use their discretion to meet the needs of individual children. Dentists were instructed not to wear white coats and not to use probes during the examination. A small hand-held torch and a mirror were allowed, although some children only co-operated without these aids. Where a child was very unwilling to co-operate, the dentist abandoned the examination, rather than upset the child.

1.4.4 The dental interview

A pilot survey carried out in May and June 1992 developed and tested the dental questionnaire. At the mainstage, the dental interview lasted approximately 20 minutes. As with the dietary survey, interviews were conducted with children's mothers if possible. The dental topics covered in relation to each child included:
- visits to the dentist and dental treatment
- toothbrushing
- the use of teething aids
- the use of bottles, dinky feeders and dummies, including the types of drinks consumed from them
- the consumption of chocolates and sweets

Respondents were also asked about any advice they had received about caring for their child's teeth and, where a child's natural parent was interviewed, they were asked briefly about their own teeth. Copies of the dental questionnaire and other survey documents are shown at Appendix B. The questionnaire for the dietary survey is also shown at Appendix B.[13]

1.5 The response

In calculating the overall level of response to the dental survey the following were taken into account:
- response at the 'sift' to identify the sample of pre-school children
- response to the dietary interview
- response to the dental recall question
- actual participation in the dental survey.

Although it was estimated that interviews on the dietary survey would be achieved in relation to about 1500 children, in the event the response was much better than anticipated and 1859 interviews were obtained. From these, permission to recall for the dental survey was obtained from 1737 parents. Interviews were subsequently achieved with 1654 parents (95% of those consenting) and 1590 children had dental examinations (92%).

Response to the dental survey is explained in more detail in Chapter 2 of this Report and response to the various elements of the dietary survey is given in Chapter 3 of the report of the diet and nutrition survey.[2]

1.6 Plan of the Report

As noted above, Chapter 2 describes response to the survey in detail. Response rates have been calculated in relation to response to the dietary survey and characteristics of the responding sample, such as social class, are compared with those of the total population of $1^{1}/_{2}$ to $4^{1}/_{2}$ year olds.

In Chapter 3 the prevalence of dental decay, shown as active or untreated decay, filled teeth, missing teeth and any decay experience, is shown for children in each age cohort of the survey. The mean number of teeth affected by different types of decay are also presented. Variations in decay between children with different background characteristics are shown.

Chapter 4 looks at the children's dental hygiene and dental care, including information on toothbrushing, visits to the dentist, dental advice received by parents and fluoride use.

Chapter 5 reports on the use of bottles, dinky feeders and dummies and presents information on the types of drinks consumed from them. As well as information from the dental interview Chapter 5 also includes information from the dietary questionnaire interview and the four-day weighed intake diary about the consumption of foods and drinks containing sugars.

Chapter 6 combines material from previous chapters in looking at variations in patterns of decay. Decay prevalence is compared for children with different patterns of dental care and dietary practices.

Chapter 7 gives results of the examinations for trauma to the incisors and erosion of the upper incisors.

Final appendices show the examination criteria (Appendix A), Interviewer fieldwork documents (Appendix B), sampling errors (Appendix F) and additional tables relating to certain chapters which are presented without comment. A summary of the dietary survey report is included as Appendix H.

Throughout the Report, all analysis is shown by age group. Male and female data are shown separately only where differences were found. Variations by social class are presented for most data. The survey was not primarily intended to provide regional analysis. Where presented, data for Scotland, Northern England, Central and South West England and Wales, London and the South East are shown separately.[14] For one key table in Chapter 3, summary figures for England and Wales are shown separately.

References and notes

[1] Department of Health and Social Security. Report on Health and Social Subjects: 10. A Nutritional Survey of pre-school children, 1967-68. HMSO (1975).

[2] Gregory J R Collins D L Davies P S W Hughes J M Clarke P C. National Diet and Nutrition Survey: children aged $1^1/_2$ to $4^1/_2$ years. Volume 1: *Report of the diet and nutrition survey*. HMSO (1995).

[3] O'Brien M. *Children's dental health in the United Kingdom 1993*. HMSO (1994).

[4] Todd J E *Children's Dental Health in England and Wales 1973* HMSO (1975).

[5] Todd J E Dodd T. *Children's dental health in the United Kingdom 1983*. HMSO (1985).

[6] Todd J E Lader D. *Adult Dental Health 1988 United Kingdom* HMSO (1991).

[7] Gray P G Todd J E. *Adult dental health in England and Wales in 1968*. HMSO (1970).

[8] Todd J E Walker A M. *Adult dental health, Volume 1, England and Wales 1968-1978*. HMSO (1980).

[9] Todd J E Walker A M, Dodd P. *Adult dental health, Volume 2, United Kingdom 1978*. HMSO (1982).

[10] Two Dental Practice Boards exist in Britain; one covers patients living in England and Wales, the other covers those living in Scotland.

[11] A child's eligibility (being aged between $1^1/_2$ and $4^1/_2$ years) was determined for the diet and nutrition survey by taking the mid-point of the fieldwork wave as the reference date of birth. Eligible dates of birth were:

wave	fieldwork dates	mid-point	eligible dates of birth
1	28.06.92 to 03.10.92	15.08.92	15.02.88 to 14.02.91
2	05.10.92 to 03.01.93	18.11.92	18.05.88 to 17.05.91
3	04.01.93 to 03.04.93	17.02.93	17.08.88 to 16.08.91
4	05.04.93 to 04.07.93	19.05.93	19.11.88 to 18.11.91

The dental examination and interview were conducted at the end of each wave of fieldwork on the diet and nutrition survey; some children will therefore have been slightly older than $4^1/_2$ years at the time of examination; these children are included in the group of those aged $3^1/_2$ to $4^1/_2$ years.

[12] 1981 census data were used as data from the 1991 census were not available when stratification took place.

[13] Data from some questions on the dietary survey questionnaire are on the dental data file. Both the dental dataset and the dietary survey database, including information not included in the initial reports will be deposited with the ESRC Data Archive at the University of Essex following publication of the reports. Independent researchers who wish to carry out their own analyses should apply to the Archive for access. For further information about archived data please contact:

Ms Kathy Sayer
ESRC Data Archive
University of Essex
Wivenhoe Park
Colchester
Essex CO4 3SQ
Great Britain

Tel: [UK] 01206 872323
Fax:[UK] 01206 872003

EMAIL: SAYEK @:ESSEX.AC.UK

[14] See Appendix G for definitions of the four 'regions' and a map.

2 Sample design, response and characteristics of respondents

2.1 Introduction

This chapter presents response rates to the dental survey and compares the characteristics of the responding sample with those of the general population of preschool children.

As the sample for the dental survey comprised respondents to the National Diet and Nutrition Survey who consented to a subsequent dental recall, the sample design and response at various stages of the dietary survey are briefly described.

2.2 The dietary survey sample

To obtain a representative sample of children aged $1^1/_2$ to $4^1/_2$ years, a postal 'sift' was undertaken involving a random stratified probability sample of 28000 addresses selected from the Post Office's Post Code Address File (PAF). The sample size for the sift was determined by:
(a) the number of preschool children required for the survey analysis and the need to have adequate numbers in each sex and age group;
(b) estimates of the proportion of households in Great Britain containing children aged $1^1/_2$ to $4^1/_2$ years from the General Household Survey,[1] taking into account likely response rates.

The sift took the form of a short postal questionnaire asking the ages of everyone living at the sampled addresses. Non-responders to the postal stage were followed up by interviewer recall and multi-household addresses identified by the postal sift were re-issued to interviewers to select one household at random. As the dietary survey had to cover possible seasonality in eating behaviour, fieldwork was carried out over a twelve month period, organised into four fieldwork waves each lasting 10 to 12 weeks; 7000 addresses were sifted at each wave. Detailed discussion of the postal and interviewer sifts is found in Appendix C of the diet and nutrition report.[2]

2.3 Response to the dietary sift

As Table 2.1 shows, total response to the postal and interviewer sifts was 93% and the sifts generated 2101 households with eligible children. The requirements of the dietary survey meant that only one eligible child per household could be included in the survey and so 2101 formed the eligible sample of preschool children whose parents were then approached regarding participation in the dietary survey.

2.4 Response to the dental survey in relation to response to the dietary survey

The dietary survey included an interview questionnaire, four-day weighed intake dietary record, measurements of height and weight, arm and head circumference, a diary of bowel movements and a blood sample. Not everyone co-operated with all elements, but all those who completed the interview were asked permission for the interviewer to return to conduct the dental survey. The recall question was asked when respondents had completed all other aspects of the dietary survey so that knowledge of the dental component would not lead to changes in the routine way mothers were feeding their children and so that response to other aspects of the survey would not be adversely affected by respondents feeling over-burdened.

Table 2.2 shows that dietary questionnaire interviews were conducted for 88% of eligible children; for 93% of these, consent to the dental recall was received. The 1737 children with consent to recall represented 83% of the eligible dietary sample of 2101. However 7% of the original sample of 25454 eligible addresses failed to reply at either the postal or interviewer sift stages and a proportion of these addresses would have contained eligible children. Assuming that the proportion of eligible children in non-responding households was the same as among responding households at the sift stages (8.9%) it can be calculated that 161 eligible children were among the non-responding addresses. The total predicted eligible sample is therefore 2262 children (2101 + 161). Taking account of all non-response, consent to the dental recall can therefore be calculated as

$$\left(\frac{1737}{2262} \right) \times 100 = 77\%$$

Table 2.1 Response to the household sifts to identify children eligible for the dietary survey

	Number of children	As % of total addresses sampled	As % of eligible addresses	As % of responding households
Total addresses sampled	**28000**	**100%**		
Ineligible addresses from postal and interviewer sifts*	2546	9%		
Eligible addresses	25454	91%	100%	
Non-contacts	835		3%	
Refusals	978		4%	
Returns	23641		93%	100%
of which:				
Households containing eligible child	**2101**		**8%**	**9%†**

* Including vacant addresses, business premises, institutions and holiday homes.
† Rounded up from 8.9%.

Table 2.2 Response to the dental survey in relation to response to the dietary survey

	Number of children children	As % of eligible dietary sample	As % of dietary interviews achieved
Eligible dietary sample	**2101**	**100%**	
Non-contacts	14	1%	
Moved	75	4%	
Refusals	153	7%	
Dietary interview achieved	1859	88%	100%
Consent to dental recall	**1737**	**83%**	**93%**
Dental examination and/or interview achieved	1658	79%	89%

It was not expected that dental interviews and examinations would be achieved for all 1737 households consenting to the recall; for example, some people would change their minds and others would move house. In the event losses were small, with dental interviews and/or examinations conducted for 1658 children. From Table 2.2 it can be seen that participants in the dental survey represented 79% of the eligible dietary sample and 89% of those for whom dietary interviews were achieved. Taking non-response at all stages including the original sifts into account the effective response to the dental survey was therefore 73%:

$$\left(\frac{1658}{2262} \right) \times 100 = 73\%$$

2.5 Response to elements of the dental survey

As described in Chapter 1, the dental survey had several elements and those participating in the dental survey did not always co-operate with all elements. In particular, dental interviews were achieved in some cases where the dental examination was refused, either by the parent or the child. In four cases the examination was completed but the interview

was refused. Table 2.3 shows that dental interviews were achieved with 95%, and examinations attempted with 92% of children for whom consent to the dental recall was achieved. The dental examination itself comprised three elements; to establish the state of the teeth (ie whether they were sound, decayed, missing or filled), to identify any trauma to incisors and to identify any erosion of the upper incisors on both the buccal (front) and palatal (back) surfaces. Not all children would tolerate all elements of the examination, resulting in some parts being omitted or only partially completed. Complete examinations and an interview were achieved for 84% of children for whom consent to recall was given (Table 2.3).

Response to the components of the examination is shown in more detail in Table 2.4. This gives the number of complete and partial examinations achieved at each stage, and the number of cases where no examination was attempted for each component. Of the children examined, a complete examination of the state of the teeth was achieved in 96% of cases; 4% of children had partial examinations. The examination for trauma involved only the front eight incisors and for 99% of children examined this component was completed. The erosion component of the examination was

Table 2.3 Response to different components of the dental survey

Response to components of dental survey	Number of children	As % of consent to dental recall
Consented to recall question	1737	100%
Examination and/or interview achieved	1658	95%
Interview achieved	1654	95%
Examination attempted*	1591	92%
Full examinations achieved†	1455	84%
Interview and full examinations achieved	1451	84%

* A complete examination for at least one component of the examination was achieved for every child where an examination was attempted.
† Children for whom complete examinations were achieved at state of the teeth, trauma to incisors and erosion of buccal and palatal surfaces of upper incisors.

Table 2.4 Response to the different components of the dental examination

Examination component	Number of children with examinations that were:			Total	Complete examinations as % of total
	complete	partial	not carried out		
State of the teeth	1532	58	1	1591	96%
Trauma to incisors	1570	12	9	1591	99%
Erosion of upper incisors					
buccal surfaces	1522	19	50	1591	96%
palatal surfaces	1496	18	77	1591	94%
All components	1455	136	0	1591	91%

carried out last and therefore was the most likely component to be omitted, however 96% and 94% of children examined had complete examinations for buccal and palatal erosion respectively. In future chapters analysis of examination data is based on full examinations for each component only and excludes information from partial examinations.

2.6 Response to elements of the survey by age and sex

This section compares responders' age and sex with general population data from the 1991 Census and OPCS Population Estimates.

Table 2.5 shows the numbers of boys and girls aged $1\frac{1}{2}$ to $2\frac{1}{2}$, $2\frac{1}{2}$ to $3\frac{1}{2}$ and $3\frac{1}{2}$ to $4\frac{1}{2}$ years co-operating with different stages of the dental survey. For each age/sex group the numbers of children where full examinations and an interview were obtained are shown as a percentage of those where interviews were obtained. Younger children were less likely to co-operate with all elements of the survey than were older children; 91% of $3\frac{1}{2}$ to $4\frac{1}{2}$ year olds had full examinations and interviews compared with 86% of children aged $1\frac{1}{2}$ to $2\frac{1}{2}$ years ($p<0.05$). Non-cooperation appears to have been slightly greater among girls than boys, but the differences are not statistically significant.

Table 2.6 compares the age and sex distributions of two response groups from the dental survey with the age and sex distributions of children interviewed on the dietary survey. The two response groups are those interviewed, and those with full examinations and interviews. A higher proportion of the dental responders than of the dietary responders were aged $3\frac{1}{2}$ to $4\frac{1}{2}$ years, and the dental sample had a correspondingly lower proportion of children aged $1\frac{1}{2}$ to $2\frac{1}{2}$ years than the dietary sample ($p<0.01$). This difference was caused by a greater drop-out rate between the dietary and dental surveys among younger children.

In the British population there are equal proportions of children aged $1\frac{1}{2}$ to $2\frac{1}{2}$, $2\frac{1}{2}$ to $3\frac{1}{2}$ and $3\frac{1}{2}$ to $4\frac{1}{2}$ years.[3] Both the dietary and dental samples were skewed slightly from this distribution, although in opposite directions. In the dental survey the proportion of children aged $1\frac{1}{2}$ to $2\frac{1}{2}$ years (30%) was smaller than the 33.3% that would be expected ($p<0.05$).

Table 2.6 Age distribution of children with dental interviews and dental interviews and full examinations, by sex compared with the dietary survey interview sample

Sex and age	Dental survey		Dietary survey interview
	Interview	Interview & full exam	
	%	%	%
Boys aged:			
$1\frac{1}{2}$ - $2\frac{1}{2}$ years	30	30	36
$2\frac{1}{2}$ - $3\frac{1}{2}$ years	37	36	35
$3\frac{1}{2}$ - $4\frac{1}{2}$ years	33	34	29
Base	*842*	*752*	*943*
Girls aged:			
$1\frac{1}{2}$ - $2\frac{1}{2}$ years	30	29	34
$2\frac{1}{2}$ - $3\frac{1}{2}$ years	36	35	37
$3\frac{1}{2}$ - $4\frac{1}{2}$ years	34	36	29
Base	*812*	*699*	*916*
All children aged:			
$1\frac{1}{2}$ - $2\frac{1}{2}$ years	30	29	35
$2\frac{1}{2}$ - $3\frac{1}{2}$ years	36	36	36
$3\frac{1}{2}$ - $4\frac{1}{2}$ years	34	35	29
All boys	**51**	**52**	**51**
All girls	**49**	**48**	**49**
Base	*1654*	*1451*	*1859*

However, the proportions aged $2\frac{1}{2}$ to $3\frac{1}{2}$ years and $3\frac{1}{2}$ to $4\frac{1}{2}$ years, 36% and 34% respectively, were not significantly greater than the proportions of children of these ages in the general population. This slight imbalance in the age distribution is unlikely to cause any serious bias in the data, since whenever there is an association with age, data from the survey are presented for the three age cohorts separately.

The responding dietary and dental samples both had slightly more boys than girls, 51% compared with 49%. Comparison with 1991 Census data[4] shows this ratio is identical to that in the general population among the ages sampled.

2.7 Main characteristics of the dental survey sample compared with the dietary survey sample and the general population.

This section describes the dental survey sample in terms of its

Table 2.5 Response to different components of the dental survey by sex and age

Survey component	Sex and age of child											
	Boys aged (in years)				Girls aged (in years)				Boys and girls aged (in years)			
	$1\frac{1}{2}$ - $2\frac{1}{2}$	$2\frac{1}{2}$ - $3\frac{1}{2}$	$3\frac{1}{2}$ - $4\frac{1}{2}$	All	$1\frac{1}{2}$ - $2\frac{1}{2}$	$2\frac{1}{2}$ - $3\frac{1}{2}$	$3\frac{1}{2}$ - $4\frac{1}{2}$	All	$1\frac{1}{2}$ - $2\frac{1}{2}$	$2\frac{1}{2}$ - $3\frac{1}{2}$	$3\frac{1}{2}$ - $4\frac{1}{2}$	All
Numbers interviewed	254	308	280	842	243	290	279	812	497	598	559	1654
Numbers with complete examination:												
state of teeth	231	288	273	792	220	256	264	740	451	544	537	1532
trauma	241	293	274	808	233	263	266	762	474	556	540	1570
buccal erosion	240	289	256	785	222	256	259	737	462	545	515	1522
palatal erosion	232	283	258	773	213	250	260	723	445	533	518	1496
Numbers with full examination and interview	223	274	255	752	203	242	254	699	426	516	509	1451
Full examination and interview as % of those interviewed	88%	89%	91%	89%	84%	83%	91%	86%	86%	86%	91%	88%

social class and regional distributions. Comparisons are made with a sub-sample of the 1992 General Household Survey [5] of 5264 households containing children aged under 5 years. Since our sample included only households with children aged 1½ to 4½ years the sub-sample of the GHS is not an exact match, however it represents a very similar group of households with young children and is the closest source of comparative data available.

2.7.1 Social class

Social class was derived from information collected on parents' occupations which was collected for both parents if present in the household. For the purposes of analysis social class of the 'head of the household' has been used throughout the Report.[6] The sample size was too small for detailed analysis by individual social classes and they have been grouped into non-manual and manual categories.

Table 2.7 compares the social class distributions for children in the dental and dietary survey samples and the GHS sub-sample. Forty four per cent of children in the dental and dietary surveys were from non-manual social class backgrounds and 52% came from the manual social class group. In 4% of cases the social class of the head of the household could not be classified. This distribution corresponds closely to the social class distribution of the general population, as identified by the GHS. There were no differences in the social class distribution of the sample by sex (table not shown).

2.7.2 Region

Dental health varies by region[7] and it is therefore very important that the sample accurately represented the regions of Great Britain. Table 2.8 shows that the distributions of the dental survey sample and the sub-sample of the 1992 GHS between four standard regions[8] are closely matched. Any apparent differences were not found to be statistically significant.

Social class distribution by region

Table 2.9 compares the social class distribution within each of the four regions for the dental interview sample and the 1992 GHS sub-sample. None of the differences between the dental sample and the GHS data is statistically significant.

2.8 Other characteristics of the dental sample

This section gives some additional information about children in the sample, including their mother's educational status, 'family type', mother's work and child care arrangements, the employment status of the head of household and whether their parents were receiving certain social security benefits. Tables are presented for the entire dental sample; that is the 1658 children who participated in the dental examination and/or interview. Checks have shown that there are no significant differences for the characteristics presented between this sample, the dental interview sample and the dental interview and full examination sample.

Table 2.7 Social class distribution of children with dental interviews, dental interviews and full examinations and dietary interviews, compared with sub-sample from the 1992 GHS

Social class	Dental survey		Dietary survey	1992 GHS sub-sample
	Interview	Interview and full exam	Interview	
	%	%	%	%
Non-manual	45	44	44	44
Manual	52	52	52	51
Unclassified	4	4	4	5
Base	*1654*	*1451*	*1859*	*5264*

Table 2.8 Regional distribution of children in the dental sample compared with the general population

Region	Dental survey		Dietary survey	1992 GHS sub-sample
	Interview	Interview and full exam	Interview	
	%	%	%	%
Scotland	10	9	10	9
Northern	25	24	25	27
Central, South West and Wales	34	35	34	33
London and South East	31	32	31	31
Base	*1654*	*1451*	*1859*	*5264*

Table 2.9 Social class distribution by region; dental sample and sub-sample from 1992 GHS compared

Region and social class	Dental interview sample	1992 GHS sub-sample
	%	%
Scotland		
Non-manual	35	42
Manual	59	53
Unclassified	6	5
Base	*164*	*468*
North		
Non-manual	38	38
Manual	58	57
Unclassified	3	5
Base	*411*	*1436*
Central, South West and Wales		
Non-manual	43	45
Manual	54	52
Unclassified	2	3
Base	*565*	*1732*
London and South East		
Non-manual	54	51
Manual	41	44
Unclassified	5	6
Base	*514*	*1628*
All regions		
Non-manual	45	44
Manual	52	51
Unclassified	4	5
Base	*1654*	*5264*

Table 2.10 Highest educational qualification of children's mothers by age of child

Mother's highest educational qualification	Age of child (in years)			
	$1^1/_2$ - $2^1/_2$	$2^1/_2$ - $3^1/_2$	$3^1/_2$ - $4^1/_2$	All ages
	%	%	%	%
Above 'A' level	19	18	17	18 ⎤ 29
GCE 'A' level	12	10	11	11 ⎦
GCE 'O' level and equivalent	37	34	34	35 ⎤ 49
CSE and equivalent*	14	15	14	14 ⎦
No qualification	18	22	23	21
Base	*497*	*601*	*560*	*1658*

* Includes 'other' qualifications.

Table 2.11 The highest educational qualification of children's mothers by social class of head of household and age of child

Mother's highest educational qualification	Age of child (in years)			
	$1^1/_2$ - $2^1/_2$	$2^1/_2$ - $3^1/_2$	$3^1/_2$ - $4^1/_2$	All ages
	%	%	%	%
Non-manual				
Above 'A' level	34	34	31	33 ⎤ 48
GCE 'A' level	16	11	18	15 ⎦
GCE 'O' level and equivalent	34	34	30	33 ⎤ 42
CSE and equivalent*	8	11	10	10 ⎦
No qualification	8	10	11	10
Base	*226*	*270*	*247*	*743*
Manual				
Above 'A' level	6	4	6	5 ⎤ 13
GCE 'A' level	7	9	6	8 ⎦
GCE 'O' level and equivalent	41	35	38	38 ⎤ 57
CSE and equivalent*	20	20	18	19 ⎦
No qualification	27	32	31	30
Base	*250*	*309*	*296*	*855*

* Includes 'other' qualifications .

2.8.1 Mothers' highest educational qualification

Table 2.10 shows the highest educational qualification of children's mothers. Overall, 29% of mothers had gained GCE 'A' levels or a higher qualification and 21% had no qualifications; the remaining 49% had other qualifications, mainly GCE 'O' levels or CSEs or GCSEs. Table 2.11 shows the distribution of mother's qualifications by the social class of the head of the household. In this Report dental topics will be analysed by social class and mother's educational qualifications independently so it is important to consider relationships between the two factors. A significantly higher proportion of mothers living in non-manual households had obtained GCE 'A' levels or higher qualifications (48%) compared with mothers living in households with a manual head (13%) (p<0.01). Mothers with no qualifications represented only 10% of those from non-manual households while representing 30% from manual social class households (p<0.01).

2.8.2 Family type

Family type describes the number of children and parents living in a household. Eighty two per cent of children in the sample lived with a married or co-habiting couple and 18% lived in households with a lone parent. *(Table 2.12)*

Table 2.12 Family type by age of child

Family type	Age of child (in years)			
	$1^1/_2$ - $2^1/_2$	$2^1/_2$ - $3^1/_2$	$3^1/_2$ - $4^1/_2$	All ages
	%	%	%	%
2 parents, 1 child	31	20	15	22 ⎤
2 parents, 2 or more children	52	63	66	61 ⎦ 82
Lone parent*, 1 child	6	7	7	7 ⎤
Lone parent*, 2 or more children	10	10	12	11 ⎦ 18
Base	*497*	*601*	*560*	*1658*

* 99% of lone parents were lone mothers.

2.8.3 Working mothers and child-care arrangements

Table 2.13 shows whether children's mothers were working at the time of interview and who looked after their children while they worked. 'Work' is defined as paid employment, in or out of the home, full or part time. For the purposes of this analysis mothers on maternity leave from their job were classified as not working at the time of interview.[9] Overall, more than half of mothers were not working (58%). Most children whose mothers did work were looked after by their fathers or other relatives while their mothers worked.

2.8.4 Employment status of head of household

Information on employment status was collected for both mothers and fathers when both were present in the household, although the employment status of the head of the household is shown throughout this Report. In 12% of cases mothers were the head of the household (table not shown).

As can be seen from Table 2.14, three-quarters of children in the dental sample lived in households where the head was working. Ten per cent of children lived in households where the head was unemployed[10] and in the remaining 15% of households the head was economically inactive[11]. Chapter 3 of the dietary survey report[2] has more information on employment status; only 6% of lone parents in the dietary sample were in employment.

2.8.5 Receipt of Benefits

Just under a third of children in the sample lived in households where the parents were receiving either Income Support or Family Credit (Table 2.15). Chapter 3 of the dietary

Table 2.13 Whether mother worked and who looked after child, by age of child

Whether mother worked and who looked after child	Age of child (in years)			
	$1^{1}/_{2}$ - $2^{1}/_{2}$	$2^{1}/_{2}$ - $3^{1}/_{2}$	$3^{1}/_{2}$ - $4^{1}/_{2}$	All ages
	%	%	%	%
Mother not working	62	57	56	58
Mother working and child looked after by:				
mother	5	5	3	4
father	12	16	13	14
other relative	11	12	13	12
paid childminder	6	5	4	5
other*	3	5	10	6
Base	*497*	*601*	*560*	*1658*

* Includes day nursery, creche, play group and nursery school.

Table 2.14 Employment status of head of household by age of child

Head of household	Age of child (in years)			
	$1^{1}/_{2}$ - $2^{1}/_{2}$	$2^{1}/_{2}$ - $3^{1}/_{2}$	$3^{1}/_{2}$ - $4^{1}/_{2}$	All ages
	%	%	%	%
Working	75	74	76	75
Unemployed	10	10	9	10
Economically inactive	15	15	15	15
Base	*497*	*601*	*560*	*1658*

Table 2.15 Whether parents in receipt of Income Support or Family Credit, by age of child

Whether parents in receipt of Income Support or Family Credit	Age of child (in years)			
	$1^{1}/_{2}$ - $2^{1}/_{2}$	$2^{1}/_{2}$ - $3^{1}/_{2}$	$3^{1}/_{2}$ - $4^{1}/_{2}$	All ages
	%	%	%	%
In receipt of Income Support or Family Credit	31	32	31	32
Not in receipt of Income Support or Family Credit	69	68	68	68
Base	*497*	*601*	*560*	*1658*

survey report[2] has more information on the characteristics of households receiving benefits; about 28% of households in the dietary sample were in receipt of Income Support and 6% were receiving Family Credit.

2.9 Conclusion

This chapter shows high response to the dental survey from the sift stages needed to identify a sample of preschool children through to participation in different elements of the dental examination. The sample of children participating in the survey accurately represents the British population aged $1^{1}/_{2}$ to $4^{1}/_{2}$ years in terms of regional distribution, social class and sex. Major characteristics of the dental sample have been described and these will later be analysed in relation to dental habits and dental health. The response analysis has shown no biases within the sample which are likely to affect the findings or necessitate weighting of the data.

References and notes

[1] It was estimated that 8.9% of households in Great Britain contained children aged $1^{1}/_{2}$ to $4^{1}/_{2}$ years; combined data from 1988/89 GHS. Breeze E Trevor G and Wilmot A. *1989 General Household Survey*. HMSO (1990).

[2] Gregory J R Collins D L Davies P S W Hughes J M Clarke P C National Diet and Nutrition Survey: children aged $1^{1}/_{2}$ to $4^{1}/_{2}$ years Volume 1: *Report of the diet and nutrition survey*. HMSO (1995) (Chapter 4).

[3] Population Estimates Unit, OPCS, Crown Copyright (Unpublished data). In mid-1992 the number of children born in 1988, 1989, 1990 and 1991 and living in Great Britain was estimated to be 3,019,644. Of these children, 25% were born in each of the four years showing an equal age distribution in the population from which our sample is drawn.

[4] *1991 Census Report for Great Britain* (Part 1) Volume 1 of 3. HMSO (1993): Table 2 'Age and Marital Status' (p64).

[5] Thomas M. Goddard E. Hickman M. Hunter P. *1992 General Household Survey* HMSO (1994).

[6] See Appendix G for definition of head of household.

[7] For example, O'Brien M.*Children's Dental Health in the United Kingdom 1993*. HMSO (1994).

[8] See Appendix G for definitions and of the four 'regions', and map.

[9] In determining the employment status of head of household, women who were the head of their household and who were on maternity leave at the time of the interview were classified as working.

[10] See Appendix G for definition of 'unemployed'.

[11] See Appendix G for definition of 'economically inactive'.

3 Condition of young children's teeth

3.1 Introduction

This chapter presents dental data for the 1532 children for whom the first component of the dental examination, 'state of the teeth', was completed. The chapter looks at measures of dental decay and discusses variations in decay levels by social class and other characteristics of children and their households; the relationships between dental habits and dental decay are discussed in Chapter 6.

3.2 Prevalence of dental decay

In the dental examination, information was recorded for each tooth to identify it as either sound, actively decayed, filled, or missing due to decay. Actively decayed teeth were defined as having decay into the dentine or pulp which was untreated at the time of the examination. Where a tooth which had erupted was missing from the mouth it was assumed to have been extracted due to decay, unless it was known to have been lost through accidental damage. The criteria used for the dental examinations are shown at Appendix A. This section shows the proportion of children with each type of decay and with any decay experience. As no differences were found for boys and girls, the data are not shown separately for the two sexes.

3.2.1 The proportion of children with active decay, filled teeth, teeth missing due to decay and with any decay experience

Overall 17% of children examined were recorded as having some decay experience (Table 3.1). The proportion varied considerably by age with only 4% of children aged $1^1/_2$ to $2^1/_2$ years having any decay experience compared with 30% of those aged $3^1/_2$ to $4^1/_2$ years (p<0.01). Most of the decay experience was untreated or 'active' decay; overall only 2% of children had had teeth filled and 2% had had teeth extracted due to decay; even among children aged $3^1/_2$ to $4^1/_2$ years the proportions with fillings and extractions only reached 4% each. (See section 3.5 for more information of the proportions of total decay experience found to be treated and untreated).

3.2.2 Variations in dental decay by characteristics of children and their households

Tables 3.2 to 3.8 show the relationships between dental decay and the social class of the head of the household, region, mother's highest educational qualification, family type, employment status of the head of household and whether children's parents were in receipt of Income Support or Family Credit; some of these variables are interrelated and associations between dental decay and each of these variables are therefore not independent. In particular, inter-relationships exist between family type, receipt of Income Support or Family Credit and the employment status of the head of household, and between the social class of the head of household and the highest educational qualifications of children's mothers (see Chapter 2 of this Report, section 2.8.1). A multi-variate analysis was carried out to identify which of the factors presented were independently associated with children having dental decay experience.[1]

The main discriminator between children with and without dental decay varied for children of different ages (see Table A). In identifying independent relationships the model first identified the variable which was most significant in explaining differences in decay experience and then controlled for the effect of this variable while selecting other variables that also discriminated between children with and without decay experience.[2] Among those aged $1^1/_2$ to $2^1/_2$ years and $2^1/_2$ to $3^1/_2$ years one main variable was identified and with this in the model, none of the other variables considered showed independent relationships with decay experience. The variables selected were for $1^1/_2$ to $2^1/_2$ year olds, whether the parents were in receipt of Income Support or Family Credit, and, for $2^1/_2$ to $3^1/_2$ year olds, the highest educational qualification of children's mothers. Among $3^1/_2$ to $4^1/_2$ year olds the social class of the head of the household was the main discriminator between children with and without dental decay. After allowing for social class, the analysis next identified region, and then whether parents were in receipt of Income Support or Family Credit, as variables independently associated with decay experience among this age group.

Table 3.1 Proportion of children with any active decay, filled teeth, teeth missing due to decay and any decay experience, by age

Type of decay	Age of child (in years)			
	$1^1/_2$ - $2^1/_2$	$2^1/_2$ - $3^1/_2$	$3^1/_2$ - $4^1/_2$	All ages
	Percentage of children with each type of decay			
Active decay	4	13	28	16
Filled teeth	-	1	4	2
Teeth missing due to decay	0	1	4	2
Any decay experience	4	14	30	17
Base	*451*	*544*	*537*	*1532*

Table A Variables which were found to be independently related to decay experience, by age, in order of importance

Age of child (in years)		
$1^1/_2$ to $2^1/_2$	$2^1/_2$ to $3^1/_2$	$3^1/_2$ to $4^1/_2$
Whether parents were in receipt of Income Support or Family Credit	Highest educational qualification of child's mother	Social class of head of household
		Region
		Whether parents were in receipt of Income Support or Family Credit

When considering the tables in this chapter, the inter-relationships outlined above should be borne in mind. The commentary for Tables 3.2 to 3.8 generally focuses on differences in total decay experience; groups with highest prevalence of decay experience tended to have highest prevalence of each of active decay, filled teeth and teeth missing due to decay. It has already been shown that most of the decay experience of young children was untreated; section 3.5 looks at treated and untreated decay in more detail and shows the proportion of total decay which was treated for children with different background characteristics.

(i) Social class of head of household

Children from manual social class backgrounds had considerably more untreated and treated dental decay than did those from non-manual backgrounds (Table 3.2). Among $3^1/_2$ to $4^1/_2$ year olds, for example, 40% of children from the manual social class group had some decay experience compared with 16% of those from households with a non-manual head (p<0.01).

(ii) Region

Scottish children and those in the North of England had more decay than those in other parts of England and Wales (Table 3.3). Half the children aged $3^1/_2$ to $4^1/_2$ years in Scotland and 43% of those in the Northern region of England had some experience of dental decay compared with less than a quarter of those in the rest of England and Wales.

A significantly higher proportion of children in Scotland than elsewhere had filled teeth. For example, among $3^1/_2$ to $4^1/_2$ year olds, 13% of Scottish children had fillings compared with 4% in the Central and South West regions of England and Wales and 3% and 2% respectively in the Northern region of England and in London and the South East (p<0.05).

Table 3.4 shows the proportions of children with each type of decay for Wales only. Although the bases are small, the data suggest that the figures for the standard region 'Central, South West and Wales' mask worse dental health in Wales

Table 3.2 Proportion of children with any active decay, filled teeth, teeth missing due to decay and any decay experience, by age and social class of head of household

Social class of head of household and type of decay	Age of child (in years)			
	$1^1/_2$ - $2^1/_2$	$2^1/_2$ - $3^1/_2$	$3^1/_2$ - $4^1/_2$	All ages
	Percentage of children with each type of decay			
Non-manual				
Active decay	3	10	15	9
Filled teeth	-	1	2	1
Teeth missing due to decay	-	0	2	1
Any decay experience	3	10	16	10
Base	*203*	*243*	*233*	*679*
Manual				
Active decay	5	17	37	21
Filled teeth	-	0	6	2
Teeth missing due to decay	0	1	5	2
Any decay experience	5	17	40	22
Base	*228*	*283*	*287*	*798*

Table 3.3 Proportion of children with any active decay, filled teeth, teeth missing due to decay and any decay experience, by age and region

Region and type of decay	Age of child (in years)			
	$1^1/_2$ - $2^1/_2$	$2^1/_2$ - $3^1/_2$	$3^1/_2$ - $4^1/_2$	All ages
	Percentage of children with each type of decay			
Scotland				
Active decay	3	18	40	23
Filled teeth	-	2	13	6
Teeth missing due to decay	-	2	8	4
Any decay experience	3	18	50	27
Base	*37*	*51*	*60*	*148*
North				
Active decay	6	15	40	20
Filled teeth	-	-	3	1
Teeth missing due to decay	1	-	4	2
Any decay experience	7	15	43	21
Base	*107*	*149*	*119*	*375*
Central, South West and Wales				
Active decay	3	10	22	12
Filled teeth	-	1	4	2
Teeth missing due to decay	-	1	3	1
Any decay experience	3	11	24	13
Base	*161*	*186*	*183*	*530*
London and South East				
Active decay	4	15	21	14
Filled teeth	-	-	2	1
Teeth missing due to decay	-	-	3	1
Any decay experience	4	15	21	14
Base	*146*	*158*	*175*	*479*

Table 3.4 Proportion of children in Wales with any active decay, filled teeth, teeth missing due to decay and any decay experience, by age

Type of decay	Age of child (in years)			
	$1^1/_2$ - $2^1/_2$	$2^1/_2$ - $3^1/_2$	$3^1/_2$ - $4^1/_2$	All ages
	Percentage of children with each type of decay			
Wales				
Active decay	-	21	37	19
Filled teeth	-	3	3	2
Teeth missing due to decay	-	3	3	2
Any decay experience	-	27	37	21
Base	*32*	*33*	*30*	*95*

than in the linked regions of England. Among Welsh children aged $3^1/_2$ to $4^1/_2$ years 37% were found to have experience of decay, a proportion closer to that of the Northern region of England than elsewhere. Data for England only are shown in Table 3.5; since most children in the survey lived in England, the proportions with each type of decay in England were similar to those for all children.

(iii) Highest educational qualification of children's mothers

Overall, experience of dental decay affected a higher proportion of children whose mothers had no educational qualifications (27%) than those whose mothers had GCE 'A' levels or a higher qualification (10%), or other lower level educational qualifications (16%) (all differences significant p<0.01).

(Table 3.6)

Table 3.5 Proportion of children in England with any active decay, filled teeth, teeth missing due to decay and any decay experience, by age

Type of decay	Age of child (in years)			
	$1^1/_2$ - $2^1/_2$	$2^1/_2$ - $3^1/_2$	$3^1/_2$ - $4^1/_2$	All ages
	Percentage of children with each type of decay			
England				
Active decay	4	12	26	15
Filled teeth	-	0	3	1
Teeth missing due to decay	0	4	3	1
Any decay experience	4	13	27	15
Base	*382*	*460*	*447*	*1289*

Table 3.6 Proportion of children with any active decay, filled teeth, teeth missing due to decay and any decay experience, by age and mother's highest educational qualification

Mother's highest educational qualification and type of decay	Age of child (in years)			
	$1^1/_2$ - $2^1/_2$	$2^1/_2$ - $3^1/_2$	$3^1/_2$ - $4^1/_2$	All ages
	Percentage of children with each type of decay			
GCE 'A' level or higher				
Active decay	2	6	18	9
Filled teeth	-	-	4	1
Teeth missing due to decay	-	1	1	1
Any decay experience	2	7	20	10
Base	*134*	*154*	*154*	*442*
Other				
Active decay	4	13	26	15
Filled teeth	-	-	4	2
Teeth missing due to decay	-	0	4	2
Any decay experience	4	14	29	16
Base	*230*	*264*	*256*	*750*
No qualifications				
Active decay	6	23	44	26
Filled teeth	-	2	5	3
Teeth missing due to decay	1	1	6	3
Any decay experience	7	24	46	27
Base	*87*	*125*	*125*	*337*

Table 3.7 Proportion of children with any active decay, filled teeth, teeth missing due to decay and any decay experience, by age and family type

Family type and type of decay	Age of child (in years)			
	$1^1/_2$ - $2^1/_2$	$2^1/_2$ - $3^1/_2$	$3^1/_2$ - $4^1/_2$	All ages
	Percentage of children with each type of decay			
Two parents and child/ children				
Active decay	4	13	26	15
Filled teeth	-	0	3	1
Teeth missing due to decay	-	0	3	1
Any decay experience	4	13	28	16
Base	*371*	*450*	*436*	*1257*
Lone parent and child/ children				
Active decay	5	16	36	20
Filled teeth	-	1	8	3
Teeth missing due to decay	1	2	8	4
Any decay experience	6	17	40	22
Base	*79*	*94*	*101*	*274*

Table 3.8 Proportion of children with any active decay, filled teeth, teeth missing due to decay and any decay experience, by age and employment status of head of household

Employment status of head of household and type of decay	Age of child (in years)			
	$1^1/_2$ - $2^1/_2$	$2^1/_2$ - $3^1/_2$	$3^1/_2$ - $4^1/_2$	All ages
	Percentage of children with each type of decay			
Working				
Active decay	2	12	23	13
Filled teeth	-	0	4	2
Teeth missing due to decay	-	0	2	1
Any decay experience	2	12	26	14
Base	*338*	*400*	*410*	*1148*
Unemployed				
Active decay	9	26	43	27
Filled teeth	-	-	4	1
Teeth missing due to decay	-	-	4	1
Any decay experience	9	26	45	27
Base	*44*	*58*	*49*	*151*
Economically inactive				
Active decay	7	14	44	22
Filled teeth	-	1	6	3
Teeth missing due to decay	1	1	10	4
Any decay experience	9	14	45	23
Base	*69*	*86*	*78*	*233*

(iv) Family type

Children living in lone-parent families were more likely than those from two-parent families to have each type of dental decay; 40% of $3^1/_2$ to $4^1/_2$ year olds from lone-parent families had some decay experience compared with 28% of those from two-parent families (p<0.05).   *(Table 3.7)*

(v) Employment status of the head of household

Table 3.8 shows a greater prevalence of dental decay experience among children from households where the head was unemployed (27% overall) or economically inactive (23%) than among those where the head of the household was working (14%) (p<0.05).

(vi) Receipt of Income Support or Family Credit

Children whose parents were in receipt of Income Support or Family Credit were more likely to have actively decayed, filled and missing teeth than those whose parents were not receiving these benefits (Table 3.9). Differences were

significant even among the youngest children; 8% of $1^1/_2$ to $2^1/_2$ year olds whose parents were in receipt of Income Support or Family Credit had experience of decay compared with 2% of those whose parents were not (p<0.05).

(vii) Social class of the head of household and receipt of Income Support or Family Credit

The multi-variate analysis for $3^1/_2$ to $4^1/_2$ year olds showed that both the social class of the head of household and whether parents were in receipt of Income Support or Family Credit were independently related to decay experience; in Table 3.10 these variables have been cross classified and their joint relationship with dental decay is presented. Vari-

13

Table 3.9 Proportion of children with any active decay, filled teeth, teeth missing due to decay and any decay experience, by age and whether parents in receipt of Income Support or Family Credit

Whether parents in receipt of Income Support or Family Credit and type of decay	Age of child (in years)			
	$1\frac{1}{2}$ - $2\frac{1}{2}$	$2\frac{1}{2}$ - $3\frac{1}{2}$	$3\frac{1}{2}$ - $4\frac{1}{2}$	All ages
	Percentage of children with each type of decay			
In receipt of benefit				
Active decay	7	19	40	23
Filled teeth	-	1	7	3
Teeth missing due to decay	1	1	7	3
Any decay experience	8	20	43	24
Base	*142*	*175*	*167*	*484*
Not in receipt of benefit				
Active decay	2	11	23	12
Filled teeth	-	1	3	1
Teeth missing due to decay	-	0	2	1
Any decay experience	2	11	25	13
Base	*309*	*369*	*369*	*1047*

Table 3.10 Proportion of children with any active decay, filled teeth, teeth missing due to decay and any decay experience, by age and social class of head of household and whether parents in receipt of Income Support or Family Credit

Social class of head of household and whether parents in receipt of Income Support or Family Credit and type of decay	Age of child (in years)			
	$1\frac{1}{2}$ - $2\frac{1}{2}$	$2\frac{1}{2}$ - $3\frac{1}{2}$	$3\frac{1}{2}$ - $4\frac{1}{2}$	All ages
	Percentage of children with each type of decay			
Non-manual, not receiving benefits				
Active decay	1	7	13	7
Filled teeth	-	1	2	1
Teeth missing due to decay	-	1	1	1
Any decay experience	1	8	14	8
Base	*170*	*196*	*191*	*557*
Non-manual, receiving benefits				
Active decay	9	19	24	18
Filled teeth	-	-	2	1
Teeth missing due to decay	0	0	7	2
Any decay experience	9	19	26	19
Base	*33*	*47*	*42*	*122*
Manual, not receiving benefits				
Active decay	3	15	33	18
Filled teeth	-	-	5	2
Teeth missing due to decay	-	-	4	1
Any decay experience	3	15	36	19
Base	*131*	*165*	*171*	*467*
Manual, receiving benefits				
Active decay	7	20	43	24
Filled teeth	-	1	9	3
Teeth missing due to decay	1	2	6	3
Any decay experience	8	20	46	26
Base	*97*	*118*	*115*	*330*

ations can be seen within both the manual and non-manual social class groups in the proportion of children with experience of dental decay, depending on whether or not the parents were in receipt of Income Support or Family Credit. Due to the small bases some of the apparent differences do not reach statistical significance, however overall a strong gradient in levels of decay can be seen. At one extreme, 46% of $3\frac{1}{2}$ to $4\frac{1}{2}$ year olds from households with a manual head, and with parents receiving Income Support or Family Credit, had some decay experience; this compares with 14% of $3\frac{1}{2}$ to $4\frac{1}{2}$ year olds from non-manual backgrounds and with parents not in receipt of Income Support or Family Credit having experience of dental decay.

(viii) Other characteristics of children and their households

Experience of dental decay was not found to be related to being the only child in a household or to being the first born child in a family as opposed to a later born child (Table 3.11). There was also no apparent difference in decay experience between children whose mothers were in paid employment and those whose mothers were not. Among children in the oldest age cohort, those who did not attend a nursery or playgroup appeared to have a higher prevalence of decay experience (43%) than children who did attend one of these (28%), but due to the small number of children not attending a nursery or playgroup this difference did not reach statistical significance (p>0.05). *(Table 3.11)*

3.2.3 Decay into the dental pulp

Most of the active decay recorded on children's teeth extended only into the dentine, but a small proportion of children in the survey, 4% overall, had decay which extended into the dental pulp (Table 3.12). Decay into the dental pulp tended to be more prevalent among groups where decay itself was more prevalent. Children whose mothers had no educational qualifications and those from households where the head was unemployed were most likely to have decay into the dental pulp although, even within these groups, only 8% of children were affected. Among $3\frac{1}{2}$ to $4\frac{1}{2}$ year olds the proportion of children with decay into the dental pulp varied notably between the areas of Britain; 17% of Scottish children of this age had some decay into the pulp compared with 12% of those in the Northern region of England and 6% or less in the rest of England and Wales (p<0.05).

While decay into the dental pulp did not affect a large proportion of children overall, of $3\frac{1}{2}$ to $4\frac{1}{2}$ year olds with some active decay, 30% had some decay which extended into the pulp (table not shown).

3.3 The number of teeth with decay experience

3.3.1 The mean number of teeth with decay experience for all children

Table 3.13 shows the mean number of teeth with active decay, treated decay, that is fillings and extractions combined, and with any experience of decay. Overall, children aged $1\frac{1}{2}$ to $2\frac{1}{2}$ years had an average of 0.1 teeth with decay experience, those aged $2\frac{1}{2}$ to $3\frac{1}{2}$ years had 0.5 teeth affected

Table 3.11 The proportion of children with any decay experience by age and the child's position in the family, whether mother did any paid work in the last week and whether child attending a nursery school or playgroup

Whether only child in the household under 16 years, whether first child, whether mother did any paid work last week and whether child attending nursery or playgroup	Age of child (in years)							
	$1^1/_2$ - $2^1/_2$		$2^1/_2$ - $3^1/_2$		$3^1/_2$ - $4^1/_2$		All ages	
	%*	Base	%*	Base	%*	Base	%*	Base
All children	4	451	14	544	30	537	17	1532
Whether only child under 16 years in household								
Only child	4	162	14	148	32	116	15	426
Not only child	4	289	14	396	30	421	17	1106
Whether mother's first born child†								
First born child	4	195	12	239	29	216	15	650
Not first born child	4	248	15	298	31	311	18	875
Whether mother did any paid work last week								
Mother worked	3	165	13	223	29	224	16	612
Mother did not work	5	286	15	320	31	312	17	918
Whether child attending nursery or playgroup								
Goes to nursery or playgroup	4	51	12	301	28	468	21	820
Does not go to nursery or playgroup	4	400	16	243	43	69	12	712

* This table shows the percentage of children with experience of decay; each percentage is calculated on the base shown in the right hand column. The column percentages do not total 100%.
† Only applied if informant was child's natural mother.

Table 3.12 Proportion of children with decay into the dental pulp by age and social class of head of household, region, mother's highest educational qualification, family type, employment status of head of household and whether parents in receipt of Income Support or Family Credit

Social class of head of household, region, mother's highest educational qualification, family type, employment status of head of household and whether parents in receipt of Income Support or Family Credit	Age of child (in years)							
	$1^1/_2$ - $2^1/_2$		$2^1/_2$ - $3^1/_2$		$3^1/_2$ - $4^1/_2$		All ages	
	%*	Base	%*	Base	%*	Base	%*	Base
All children	0	451	3	544	8	537	4	1532
Social class of head of household								
Non-manual	-	203	4	243	5	233	3	679
Manual	0	228	3	283	11	287	5	798
Region								
Scotland	-	37	-	51	17	60	7	148
North	1	107	5	149	12	119	6	375
Central, South West and Wales	-	161	3	186	6	183	3	530
London and South East	0	146	3	158	5	175	3	479
Mother's highest educational qualification								
'A' level or higher	-	134	1	154	5	154	2	442
Other	0	230	3	264	7	256	4	750
None	-	87	6	125	14	125	8	337
Family type								
Two parents and child/ children	-	371	3	450	8	436	4	1257
Lone parent and child/ children	1	79	3	94	9	101	5	274
Employment status of head of household								
Working	-	338	3	400	7	410	3	1148
Unemployed	-	44	10	58	12	49	8	151
Economically inactive	0	69	1	86	14	78	6	233
Parents receiving benefit?								
Yes	1	142	5	175	13	167	6	484
No	-	309	3	369	6	369	3	1047

* This table shows the percentage of children with experience of decay into the dental pulp; each percentage is calculated on the base shown in the right hand column. The column percentages do not total 100%.

and an average of 1.3 teeth showed decay experience among those in the oldest age cohort. Fillings and extractions were only evident among children aged $3^1/_2$ to $4^1/_2$ years where an average of 0.3 teeth had been treated for caries in addition to 1.0 teeth on average having active decay. Due to the generally low levels of treated decay, the rest of this section refers only to decay experience and not to its various components.

Children living in Scotland and those whose mothers had no educational qualifications had the highest mean number of teeth with decay experience (Table 3.14). For example, Scottish children aged $3^1/_2$ to $4^1/_2$ years had an average of 2.4 affected teeth and children of the same age whose mothers had no educational qualifications had an average of 2.2

affected teeth. Children whose mothers had GCE 'A' levels or higher qualifications had the lowest mean number of teeth with decay experience (0.3 teeth affected overall).

3.3.2 The mean number of teeth with experience of decay for children with some decayed teeth

In previous sections the proportion of children with dental decay has been shown to vary according to certain background characteristics. This section aims to identify whether background characteristics explained different levels of dental decay, considering just those with some decay experience. Caries prevalence was too low among younger children for this further analysis, so data are presented only for those aged $3^1/_2$ to $4^1/_2$ years; for $3^1/_2$ to $4^1/_2$ year olds with some decay experience, means of 3.3 actively decayed teeth and 0.9 filled or extracted teeth were recorded (table not shown).

Table 3.15 shows that the mean number of teeth with decay experience for $3^1/_2$ to $4^1/_2$ year olds with some decay experience was 4.2. The data suggest that children with decay, from groups with higher decay prevalence, (for example Scottish children and those whose mothers had no educational qualifications), generally had more teeth affected by decay than those with decay from groups with lower decay prevalence (for example children whose mothers had GCE 'A' levels or higher qualifications and those from households where the head was employed). However, due to the small bases, apparent variations in the data do not reach levels of statistical significance.

Table 3.13   The mean number of teeth with active decay, evidence of treatment (filled or missing teeth) and any decay experience, by age

Type of decay	Age of child (in years)			
	$1^1/_2$ - $2^1/_2$	$2^1/_2$ - $3^1/_2$	$3^1/_2$ - $4^1/_2$	All ages
	The mean number of teeth with each type of decay			
Active decay	0.1	0.4	1.0	0.5
Filled or missing teeth	0	0	0.3	0.1
Any decay experience	0.1	0.5	1.3	0.6
Base	*451*	*544*	*537*	*1532*

Table 3.14   The mean number of teeth with any decay experience by age and social class of head of household, region, mother's highest educational qualification, family type, employment status of head of household and whether parents in receipt of Income Support or Family Credit

Social class of head of household, region, mother's highest educational qualification, family type, employment status of head of household and whether parents in receipt of Income Support or Family Credit	Age of child (in years)							
	$1^1/_2$ - $2^1/_2$		$2^1/_2$ - $3^1/_2$		$3^1/_2$ - $4^1/_2$		All ages	
	Mean	*Base*	Mean	*Base*	Mean	*Base*	Mean	*Base*
All children	0.1	*451*	0.5	*544*	1.3	*537*	0.6	*1532*
Social class of head of household								
Non-manual	0	*203*	0.4	*243*	0.6	*233*	0.4	*679*
Manual	0.1	*228*	0.6	*283*	1.7	*287*	0.8	*798*
Region								
Scotland	0	*37*	0.5	*51*	2.4	*60*	1.2	*148*
North	0.2	*107*	0.6	*149*	1.5	*119*	0.8	*375*
Central, South West and Wales	0	*161*	0.4	*186*	1.0	*183*	0.5	*530*
London and South East	0.1	*146*	0.4	*158*	1.0	*175*	0.5	*479*
Mother's highest educational qualification								
'A' level or higher	0	*134*	0.2	*154*	0.7	*154*	0.3	*442*
Other	0.1	*230*	0.5	*264*	1.1	*256*	0.6	*750*
None	0.2	*87*	0.8	*125*	2.2	*125*	1.2	*337*
Family type								
Two parents and child/children	0.1	*371*	0.4	*450*	1.1	*436*	0.6	*1257*
Lone parent and child/children	0.2	*79*	0.6	*94*	2.0	*101*	1.0	*274*
Employment status of head of household								
Working	0.1	*338*	0.4	*400*	0.9	*410*	0.5	*1148*
Unemployed	0.2	*44*	1.0	*58*	1.9	*49*	1.0	*151*
Economically inactive	0.2	*69*	0.5	*86*	2.6	*78*	1.1	*233*
Parents receiving benefit?								
Yes	0.2	*142*	0.7	*175*	2.1	*167*	1.0	*484*
No	0	*309*	0.4	*369*	0.9	*369*	0.5	*1047*

Table 3.15 The mean number of teeth with any decay experience, for children aged 3¹/₂ - 4¹/₂ years with some decay experience by age and social class of head of household, region, mother's highest educational qualification, family type, employment status of head of household and whether parents in receipt of Income Support or Family Credit

Social class of head of household, region, mother's highest educational qualification, family type, employment status of head of household and whether parents in receipt of Income Support or Family Credit	Age of child (in years)	
	3¹/₂ - 4¹/₂	
	Mean	Base
All children	4.2	162
Social class of head of household		
Non-manual	3.9	37
Manual	4.2	115
Region		
Scotland	4.9	30
North	3.5	51
Central, South West and Wales	4.1	44
London and South East	4.5	37
Mother's highest educational qualification		
'A' level or higher	3.5	30
Other	3.9	75
None	4.9	57
Family type		
Two parents and child/ children	3.9	122
Lone parent and child/ children	4.9	40
Employment status of head of household		
Working	3.6	105
Unemployed	[4.2]	22
Economically inactive	5.8	35
Parents receiving benefit?		
Yes	4.8	71
No	3.6	91

Table 3.16 The number of teeth with decay experience by age

Number of teeth with decay experience	Age of child (in years)			
	1¹/₂ - 2¹/₂	2¹/₂ - 3¹/₂	3¹/₂ - 4¹/₂	All ages
	Cum %	Cum %	Cum %	Cum %
0	96	86	70	83
1	98	90	77	88
2	98	93	84	91
3	99	95	87	93
4	100*	96	90	95
5		97	92	96
6		98	94	97
7		99	95	98
8		99	96	98
9		100†	97	99
10 - 16			100	100
Range in number of teeth with decay experience	0-6	0-14	0-16	0-16
Base	*451*	*544*	*537*	*1532*

* Due to rounding, 100% of children are recorded as having no more than 4 teeth with decay experience although one child in fact had 6 teeth affected.

† Due to rounding, 100% of children are recorded as having no more than 9 teeth with decay experience although three children in fact had 10 or more teeth affected.

3.3.4 Decay into the dental pulp

Overall children in the survey had an average of 0.1 teeth with decay into the dental pulp. Of those with some decay experience an average of 0.7 teeth had decay into the dental pulp while of those with some decay into the pulp, the mean number of teeth affected was 2.9. *(Table 3.17)*

3.4 Decay on molars, incisors and canines

Table 3.18 shows which teeth were recorded as having active decay or any decay experience for children of different ages. More children had decay experience on molars (13%) than on incisors (8%) or canines (1%) (p<0.01).

For children aged 3¹/₂ to 4¹/₂ years with some decay experience, 89% had decay on their molars, 44% had decay on their incisors and 8% had decay on their canines (Table 3.19). The proportion with decay experience on molars did not vary greatly by different characteristics; more variation was apparent with regard to decay of the incisors. As the bases are small for this group, apparent differences did not reach statistical significance, however given a larger sample it is likely that some of the more substantial differences would have registered as significant; for example, among 3¹/₂ to 4¹/₂ year olds with some decay experience 40% of those from

3.3.3 The range in the number of teeth with decay experience

Table 3.16 shows the proportions of children with different numbers of teeth affected by decay. The first row shows the percentage of children with no decay experience and subsequent rows show how the percentages increase when children with one, two, three etc teeth with decay experience are included. For example, among 1¹/₂ to 2¹/₂ year olds, 98% of children had one tooth or fewer with experience of decay while among those aged 3¹/₂ to 4¹/₂ years, only 77% had decay in no more than one tooth. Among 3¹/₂ to 4¹/₂ year olds, the 10% of children with most decay experience had 4 or more teeth affected; children aged 2¹/₂ to 3¹/₂ years with only one tooth with decay experience were among the 10% of that age group with most decay. The maximum number of teeth affected by decay ranged from 6 among children aged 1¹/₂ to 2¹/₂ years to 16 among children aged 3¹/₂ to 4¹/₂ years.

Table 3.17 The mean number of teeth with decay into the dental pulp by age, for all children, those with any decay and those with any decay into the dental pulp

Level of decay experience	Age of child (in years)							
	1¹/₂ - 2¹/₂		2¹/₂ - 3¹/₂		3¹/₂ - 4¹/₂		All ages	
	Mean	Base	Mean	Base	Mean	Base	Mean	Base
All children	0	451	0.1	544	0.2	537	0.1	1532
Children with some decay experience	[0.2]	18	0.7	76	0.8	162	0.7	256
Children with some decay into the dental pulp	[0]	1	[2.8]	18	2.9	44	2.9	63

17

two-parent families had decayed incisors compared with 58% of those from lone-parent families.

Table 3.18 Proportion of children with any active decay and decay experience on molars, incisors and canines, by age

Tooth type and type of decay	Age of child (in years)			
	1½ - 2½	2½ - 3½	3½ - 4½	All ages
	Percentage of children with each type of decay			
Molars				
Active decay	2	9	24	12
Any decay experience	2	10	27	13
Incisors				
Active decay	2	7	12	7
Any decay experience	2	8	13	8
Canines				
Active decay	-	1	2	1
Any decay experience	0	1	2	1
Base	*451*	*544*	*537*	*1532*

Table 3.19 Proportion of children with any decay experience on molars, incisors and canines for children aged 3½ - 4½ years with some decay experience by age and social class of head of household, region, mother's highest educational qualification, family type, employment status of head of household and whether parents in receipt of Income Support or Family Credit

Social class of head of household, region, mother's highest ecucational qualification, family type, employment status of head of household and whether parents in receipt of Income Support or Family Credit	Tooth type			
	Molars	Incisors	Canines	Base
	*Percentage of children with decay experience**			*Base*
All children aged 3½ - 4½ years	89	44	8	*162*
Social class of head of household				
Non-manual	89	38	11	*37*
Manual	90	46	8	*115*
Region				
Scotland	90	47	10	*30*
North	90	37	2	*51*
Central, South West and Wales	86	50	7	*44*
London and South East	89	46	16	*37*
Mother's highest educational qualification				
'A' level or higher	97	30	3	*30*
Other	81	49	9	*75*
None	95	46	9	*57*
Family type				
Two parents and child/ children	89	40	7	*122*
Lone parent and child/ children	90	58	10	*40*
Employment status of head of household				
Working	86	41	7	*105*
Unemployed	[91]	[41]	[5]	*22*
Economically inactive	97	57	14	*35*
Parents receiving benefit?				
Yes	89	52	10	*71*
No	89	39	7	*91*

* All percentages are calculated on the base in the far right column.

18

3.5 Treatment of decay

Most of the decay experience among preschool children has been shown to be active or untreated decay. Table 3.20 shows the proportion of decay experience across all children in the sample which had been treated, either through filling or extracting teeth. The proportions were calculated by dividing the total number of filled or extracted teeth in all mouths in the sample by the total number of teeth with experience of decay. Overall 17% of teeth with caries experience had been filled or extracted; active decay was found on the remaining 83% of decayed teeth. Among children in the oldest age cohort a greater proportion of carious teeth had been treated (22%) than among children aged 1½ to 2½ years (10%) (p<0.05) and 2½ to 3½ years (6%) (p<0.01).

Table 3.20 Proportion of dental decay which was treated and untreated among children in the survey, by age

Type of decay	Age of child (in years)			
	1½ - 2½	2½ - 3½	3½ - 4½	All ages
	%	%	%	%
Treated decay	10	6	22	17
Untreated decay	90	94	78	83
*Base**	*42*	*256*	*673*	*971*

* The base represents the total number of carious teeth across all children who were recorded as having experience of caries.

Table 3.21 shows the proportion of decayed teeth which had been treated by filling or extracting the tooth for children with different background characteristics. Overall the most significant variation was found by region; in Scotland, a higher proportion of decay (28%) was treated than in the North of England (10%, p<0.01) or the rest of England and Wales (17%, p<0.05). Treated decay also represented a significantly higher proportion of total decay among children from two-parent families (25%) than among those from lone-parent families (11%) (p<0.01). Other apparent differences in Table 3.21 were not found to be statistically significant.

3.6 Distribution of tooth conditions around the mouth

This chapter has described the prevalence of dental decay and given an indication of which types of teeth were most likely to be affected. Figure 1 shows the proportion of children with different conditions recorded for each tooth. That is, the proportion of children for whom each individual tooth was found to be unerupted, sound, actively decayed, filled or missing.

For more than half the children aged 1½ to 2½ years the second deciduous molars in each jaw had not erupted. Eleven per cent of children in this age group were also missing their canines and a small proportion of children had unerupted first molars (2%) and second incisors (1%, lower jaw only). Decay levels were very low with the upper incisors most likely to be affected; the small amount of decay in the bottom jaw was found on the first molars.

By the age of 2½ to 3½ years all of the teeth were erupted except for the second deciduous molars in 6% of cases (upper

Table 3.21 Proportion of dental decay which was treated among children of different ages, by social class of head of household, region, mother's highest educational qualification, family type, employment status of head of household and whether parents were in receipt of Income Support or Family Credit

Social class of head of household, region, mother's highest educational qualification, family type, employment status of head of household and whether parents in receipt of Income Support or Family Credit	Age of child (in years)							
	1½ - 2½		2½ - 3½		3½ - 4½		All ages	
	%	Base	%	Base	%	Base	%	Base
All children	10	42	6	256	22	673	17	971
Social class of head of household								
Non-manual	[0]	8	11	92	28	145	21	245
Manual	13	31	4	162	21	484	16	677
Region								
Scotland	[0]	1	[4]	25	30	146	28	172
North	[4]	22	-	85	13	180	10	287
Central, South West and Wales	[0]	7	15	78	19	180	17	265
London and South East	[0]	12	-	68	26	167	17	247
Mother's highest educational qualification								
'A' level or higher	[0]	2	[1]	25	27	105	22	132
Other	[0]	23	2	128	24	289	16	440
None	[4]	17	13	103	17	279	16	399
Family type								
Two parents and child/children	[0]	6	22	45	27	129	25	180
Lone parent and child/children	[0]	17	-	150	16	347	11	514
Employment status of head of household								
Working	[0]	18	8	155	20	379	16	552
Unemployed	[0]	7	-	59	12	92	7	158
Economically inactive	[4]	17	10	42	28	202	25	261
Parents receiving benefit?								
Yes	13	30	5	122	21	344	17	496
No	[0]	12	7	134	22	329	17	475

* This table shows the percentage of total decay which was treated; each percentage is calculated on the base shown in the right hand column. The column percentages do not total 100%.

† The base represents the total number of carious teeth across all children who were recorded as having experience of caries.

jaw) and 5% of cases (lower jaw). Each tooth on the top jaw and the deciduous molars on the bottom jaw were affected by active decay for a small proportion of children.

Between the ages of 2½ to 3½ years and 3½ to 4½ years there was an increase in decay on the lower deciduous molars so that these teeth were the most likely to be decayed among 3½ to 4½ year olds. There was also evidence of some treated decay among the oldest children that was not found for 2½ to 3½ year olds, although only a small proportion of children had decay which had been treated. Treatment varied on different teeth; on the deciduous molars, fillings had been used, while the upper incisors had been extracted where any treatment had been received.

References and notes

[1] Logistic regression was used to produce a multi-variate model, with a forward stepwise method. All the variables were categorical and the dependent variable was dichotomous, recording whether or not children had experience of dental decay.

[2] All variables selected by the model had differences in decay experience between categories which were significant at the 95% level (p<0.05). The first variable to be selected by the model was the one which had the highest significance value. Additional variables had to meet the criteria of differences significant at the 95% level, with the effect of variables already in the model being controlled for. The logistic regression only identified relationships in priority order; the strengths of the independent associations cannot be obtained from this technique.

Figure 3.1 The distribution of tooth conditions around the mouth, by age

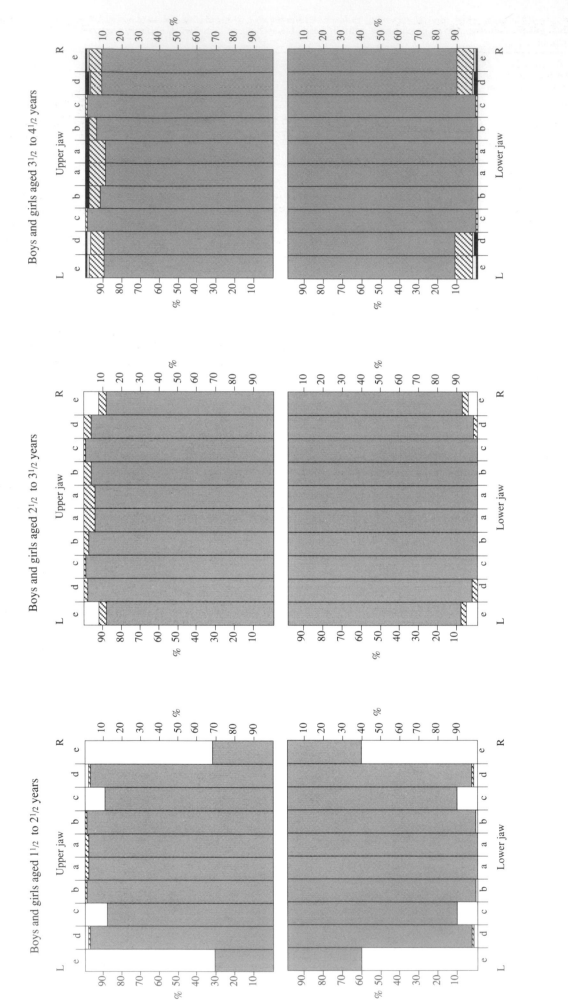

Boys and girls aged 1½ to 2½ years

Boys and girls aged 2½ to 3½ years

Boys and girls aged 3½ to 4½ years

Condition of deciduous teeth

unerupted   extracted   filled   actively decayed   sound

'e' = second deciduous molar   'd' = first deciduous molar   'c' = canine   'b' = lateral incisor   'a' = central incisor

4 Dental care and advice

4.1 Introduction

This chapter is based on information collected during the dental interview and looks at children's dental experiences including teething, dental examinations and toothbrushing, and at advice received by parents on dental health. The data analysis and hence the structure of many of the tables in this chapter was determined by the way in which the questions were asked during the interview. A copy of the questionnaire is shown at Appendix B.

4.2 Visits to a dentist

Parents were asked whether their child had ever seen a dentist prior to the dental survey, with a distinction made between visiting the dentist and being examined, and visiting the dentist just to get used to going. A quarter of $1^1/_2$ to $2^1/_2$ year olds, half the children aged $2^1/_2$ to $3^1/_2$ years and three quarters of those aged $3^1/_2$ to $4^1/_2$ years had been examined.

(Table 4.1)

A greater proportion of children from manual than from non-manual home backgrounds had never seen a dentist; for example, among $1^1/_2$ to $2^1/_2$ year olds 72% of children from manual households had never seen a dentist compared with 60% of those from non-manual backgrounds (p<0.05). Among $3^1/_2$ to $4^1/_2$ year olds 72% of children from manual households had been examined compared with 82% from non-manual households (p<0.05). *(Table 4.2)*

Children in Scotland were less likely to have been examined by a dentist than those in other regions, with the differences particularly evident in the younger two age cohorts. *(Table 4.3)*

Children whose mothers had no qualifications were considerably less likely (p<0.01) to have been examined by a dentist than those whose mothers had a qualification. The level of qualification did not have a great effect; variations between the children of mothers with GCSE and equivalent ('other') qualifications and those with GCE 'A' levels or higher qualifications were statistically significant (p<0.05) only among children in the oldest age group ($3^1/_2$ to $4^1/_2$ years). *(Table 4.4)*

Children's experiences of visiting the dentist were strongly related to the dental attendance patterns of their mothers (see section 4.7).

4.3 Advice received by parents on dental care issues

Respondents were asked whether they had ever had advice about what their child should be eating and drinking to look after their teeth and about cleaning their child's teeth. They were also asked two questions about receiving advice to give, or not to give, their child fluoride supplements in tablet or drop form,[1] and they were asked who had given any advice. More than one source could be named.

Table 4.1 Visits to the dentist by age of child

Experience of the dentist	Age of child (in years)			
	$1^1/_2$ - $2^1/_2$	$2^1/_2$ - $3^1/_2$	$3^1/_2$ - $4^1/_2$	All ages
	%	%	%	%
Seen and examined by a dentist	24	51	76	52
Seen but not examined by dentist	9	9	4	7
Never seen by a dentist	67	40	20	41
Base	*497*	*598*	*559*	*1654*

Table 4.2 Visits to the dentist by social class of head of household and age of child

Social class of head of household and visits to the dentist	Age of child (in years)			
	$1^1/_2$ - $2^1/_2$	$2^1/_2$ - $3^1/_2$	$3^1/_2$ - $4^1/_2$	All ages
	%	%	%	%
Non - manual				
Seen and examined by dentist	27	55	82	56
Seen but not examined by dentist	12	10	4	9
Never seen by dentist	60	35	14	36
Base	*226*	*268*	*246*	*740*
Manual				
Seen and examined by dentist	22	49	72	49
Seen but not examined by dentist	6	7	5	6
Never seen by dentist	72	44	23	45
Base	*250*	*308*	*296*	*854*

Table 4.3 Visits to the dentist by region and age of child

Region and visits to the dentist	Age of child (in years)			
	$1^1/_2$ - $2^1/_2$	$2^1/_2$ - $3^1/_2$	$3^1/_2$ - $4^1/_2$	All ages
	%	%	%	%
Scotland				
Seen and examined by dentist	16	39	72	46
Seen but not examined by dentist	9	7	5	7
Never seen by dentist	75	54	23	48
Base	*44*	*56*	*64*	*164*
North				
Seen and examined by dentist	28	51	76	52
Seen but not examined by dentist	7	10	5	7
Never seen by dentist	64	40	19	41
Base	*118*	*168*	*125*	*411*
Central, South West and Wales				
Seen and examined by dentist	28	58	73	54
Seen but not examined by dentist	8	6	4	6
Never seen by dentist	64	36	23	40
Base	*173*	*202*	*190*	*565*
London and South East				
Seen and examined by dentist	19	48	81	51
Seen but not examined by dentist	12	11	4	9
Never seen by dentist	69	41	14	41
Base	*162*	*172*	*180*	*514*

Table 4.4 Visits to the dentist by mother's highest educational qualification and age of child

Mother's highest educational qualification and visits to the dentist	Age of child (in years)			
	$1^1/_2$ - $2^1/_2$	$2^1/_2$ - $3^1/_2$	$3^1/_2$ - $4^1/_2$	All ages
	%	%	%	%
GCE 'A' level or higher				
Seen and examined by dentist	26	55	85	56
Seen but not examined by dentist	13	13	6	11
Never seen by dentist	61	32	9	34
Base	*152*	*167*	*159*	*478*
Other				
Seen and examined by dentist	26	54	76	53
Seen but not examined by dentist	9	8	3	7
Never seen by dentist	66	38	19	40
Base	*254*	*298*	*267*	*819*
No qualifications				
Seen and examined by dentist	18	40	63	43
Seen but not examined by dentist	3	5	5	4
Never seen by dentist	79	55	32	53
Base	*91*	*132*	*131*	*354*

Table 4.6 Advice on dental care received by parents by social class of head of household and age of child

Social class of head of household and type of advice	Age of child (in years)			
	$1^1/_2$ - $2^1/_2$	$2^1/_2$ - $3^1/_2$	$3^1/_2$ - $4^1/_2$	All ages
	Percentage of parents receiving advice			
Non-manual				
Food and drink	49	43	50	47
Teeth cleaning	29	29	41	33
Giving fluoride	26	27	30	28
Not giving fluoride	14	14	13	14
None of the above	38	35	26	33
Base	*226*	*268*	*246*	*740*
Manual				
Food and drink	34	36	42	37
Teeth cleaning	19	28	33	27
Giving fluoride	18	18	19	18
Not giving fluoride	4	6	6	6
None of the above	50	45	42	45
Base	*250*	*308*	*296*	*854*

4.3.1 Type of advice

Sixty per cent of parents had received advice on at least one of the aspects of dental care asked about (Table 4.5). More parents had received advice on what children should be eating and drinking (41%) than on the other issues. Just under a quarter of parents had received advice to give their child fluoride supplements and just less than one in ten had received advice not to give their child fluoride drops or tablets. Overall 42% of parents who had received advice not to give fluoride had also received advice to give fluoride (table not shown). (The use of fluoride toothpaste and of fluoride supplements is discussed in section 4.6).

Parents from non-manual households were more likely to report having received advice on all topics than those from manual households. *(Table 4.6)*

Parents of children in Scotland were far more likely (p<0.01) than those in other countries to have been advised to give their child fluoride drops or tablets. Sixty five per cent of Scottish parents had received this advice compared with 24% in London and the South East, 18% in the Northern region and 12% in the Central and South West regions of England, and Wales. *(Table 4.7)*

Table 4.5 Advice on dental care received by parents, by age of child

Type of advice	Age of child (in years)			
	$1^1/_2$ - $2^1/_2$	$2^1/_2$ - $3^1/_2$	$3^1/_2$ - $4^1/_2$	All ages
	Percentage of parents receiving advice			
Food and drink	40	39	45	41
Teeth cleaning	24	29	37	30
Giving fluoride	21	22	24	23
Not giving fluoride	9	10	9	9
None of the above	45	40	35	40
Base	*497*	*598*	*559*	*1654*

Table 4.7 Advice on dental care received by parents, by region and age of child

Region and type of advice	Age of child (in years)			
	$1^1/_2$ - $2^1/_2$	$2^1/_2$ - $3^1/_2$	$3^1/_2$ - $4^1/_2$	All ages
	Percentage of parents receiving advice			
Scotland				
Food and drink	43	32	53	43
Teeth cleaning	23	32	39	32
Giving fluoride	71	64	63	65
Not giving fluoride	9	7	8	8
None of the above	16	21	25	21
Base	*44*	*56*	*64*	*164*
North				
Food and drink	37	36	47	40
Teeth cleaning	24	27	38	29
Giving fluoride	17	16	20	18
Not giving fluoride	8	7	6	7
None of the above	51	50	32	45
Base	*118*	*168*	*125*	*411*
Central, South West and Wales				
Food and drink	42	44	44	43
Teeth cleaning	23	29	35	29
Giving fluoride	13	13	10	12
Not giving fluoride	6	11	6	8
None of the above	47	39	41	42
Base	*173*	*202*	*190*	*565*
London and South East				
Food and drink	40	39	43	40
Teeth cleaning	25	29	37	31
Giving fluoride	19	25	28	24
Not giving fluoride	14	13	14	14
None of the above	46	39	33	39
Base	*162*	*172*	*180*	*514*

4.3.2 Source of advice

Dentists and dental ancillaries (including dental nurses, hygienists, therapists and assistants) were the main source of advice on all issues to do with dental care; over 40% of those receiving advice on each topic were advised by dentists or dental ancillaries and 73% of teeth-cleaning advice came from this source. The other major sources of advice were health visitors and health clinics, followed by books and leaflets. *(Table 4.8)*

4.4 Teething

4.4.1 Degree of difficulty teething

Parents were asked to compare the teething experiences of their child with those of other children and assess whether their child had had 'no', 'little', 'some' or 'a lot' of difficulty teething. This scale could obviously be perceived differently by parents and a 'memory effect' is suggested by a greater proportion of older than of younger children being said to

have had no difficulty teething. Forty three per cent of all children were reported to have had no difficulty teething although among those aged $1^1/_2$ to $2^1/_2$ years only one third were reported to have had no difficulty teething. Six per cent of children were reported to have had a lot of difficulty teething and this was fairly consistent across all age groups. *(Table 4.9)*

4.4.2 Use of teething aids

Ninety per cent of children in the survey had used some type of teething aid. The most popular teething aids were 'balm or gel', used by 68% of children, and 'medicine or painkillers', used by 63%[2] (Table 4.10). The use of teething aids increased with the degree of difficulty children had teething; for example, medicines or painkillers were used by 93% of children reported to have had a lot of difficulty teething, 85% of those said to have had some difficulty teething, 70% of those regarded as having little difficulty and only 44% of those who were said to have had no difficulty teething. *(Table 4.11)*

Table 4.8 Sources of advice for parents who received advice on aspects of dental care, by age of child

Types and sources of advice	Age of child (in years)			
	$1^1/_2$ - $2^1/_2$	$2^1/_2$ - $3^1/_2$	$3^1/_2$ - $4^1/_2$	All ages
	Percentage of parents receiving advice			
Food and drink				
Dentist/dental nurse *	33	45	57	46
Health visitor to home	27	26	19	24
Child health clinic†	26	18	17	20
Friend/relative	6	10	6	7
Books/leaflets	30	28	24	27
Television	5	9	4	6
Other§	1	3	3	2
Base	*200*	*233*	*253*	*686*
Teeth cleaning				
Dentist/dental nurse*	58	74	80	73
Health visitor to home	17	8	5	9
Child health clinic†	15	9	7	10
Friend/relative	3	3	0	2
Books/leaflets	15	13	13	14
Television	2	2	1	2
Other§	3	3	2	3
Base	*118*	*172*	*205*	*495*
Giving fluoride				
Dentist/dental nurse*	41	42	48	44
Health visitor to home	30	39	27	32
Child health clinic†	26	21	29	25
Friend/relative	3	2	2	2
Books/leaflets	3	2	-	1
Other§	1	2	2	2
Base	*105*	*133*	*135*	*373*
Not giving fluoride				
Dentist/dental nurse*	44	42	52	46
Health visitor to home	16	15	14	15
Child health clinic†	20	12	6	12
Friend/relative	11	15	10	12
Books/leaflets	7	12	8	9
Television	7	5	8	6
Other§	4	7	6	6
Base	*45*	*59*	*50*	*154*

* Including advice from a dental hygienist, therapist or assistant.
† Including advice from a doctor or dietician, a nurse or midwife in hospital and advice from a mother and baby or parentcraft class.
§ Including advice from a chemist or other shop.

Table 4.9 Teething difficulties by sex and age of child

Teething difficulties	Age of child (in years)			
	$1^1/_2$ - $2^1/_2$	$2^1/_2$ - $3^1/_2$	$3^1/_2$ - $4^1/_2$	All ages
	%	%	%	%
Boys				
No difficulty	36	43	48	43
Little difficulty	34	34	30	33
Some difficulty	21	18	15	18
Lot of difficulty	8	5	7	7
Base	*254*	*308*	*280*	*842*
Girls				
No difficulty	29	46	53	44
Little difficulty	37	32	31	33
Some difficulty	27	20	11	19
Lot of difficulty	7	3	4	4
Base	*243*	*290*	*279*	*812*
Boys and girls				
No difficulty	33	44	51	43
Little difficulty	36	33	31	33
Some difficulty	24	19	13	18
Lot of difficulty	7	4	6	6
Base	*497*	*598*	*559*	*1654*

Table 4.10 Type of teething aids used by age of child

Teething aid used	Age of child (in years)			
	$1^1/_2$ - $2^1/_2$	$2^1/_2$ - $3^1/_2$	$3^1/_2$ - $4^1/_2$	All ages
	*Percentage of children**			
Balm or gel	68	69	67	68
Medicine or painkillers	71	61	58	63
Teething ring	54	51	55	53
Special biscuits/rusks	29	27	30	29
Other†	13	9	8	10
No teething aids used	7	10	10	9
Base	*497*	*598*	*559*	*1654*

* Percentages add to more than 100% as some children used more than one type of teething aid.
† Including teething granules and powders, alcohol and ice-cubes.

23

Table 4.11 Teething difficulties and type of teething aids used by age of child

Teething difficulties and teething aids used	Age of child (in years)			
	$1^1/_2$ - $2^1/_2$	$2^1/_2$ - $3^1/_2$	$3^1/_2$ - $4^1/_2$	All ages
	*Percentage of children **			
No difficulty teething				
Balm or gel	50	58	57	56
Medicine or painkillers	48	44	42	44
Teething ring	47	45	48	47
Special biscuits/rusks	20	22	26	23
Other†	9	5	6	6
No teething aids used	18	17	15	16
Base	*163*	*265*	*283*	*711*
Little difficulty teething				
Balm or gel	75	75	71	74
Medicine or painkillers	78	65	69	70
Teething ring	53	51	60	55
Special biscuits/rusks	29	27	29	29
Other†	11	10	7	10
No teething aids used	3	6	4	4
Base	*178*	*197*	*172*	*547*
Some difficulty teething				
Balm or gel	76	83	83	80
Medicine or painkillers	84	87	83	85
Teething ring	63	57	61	60
Special biscuits/rusks	35	32	42	35
Other†	19	13	11	15
No teething aids used	1	3	3	2
Base	*119*	*112*	*72*	*303*
Lot of difficulty teething				
Balm or gel	84	[21]	100	90
Medicine or painkillers	100	[22]	87	93
Teething ring	51	[18]	71	64
Special biscuits/rusks	43	[13]	45	47
Other†	11	[6]	19	17
No teething aids used	-	[-]	0	0
Base	*37*	*24*	*31*	*92*

* Percentages add to more than 100% as some children used more than one type of teething aid.
† Including teething granules and powders, alcohol and ice-cubes.

Those from the manual social classes were generally more likely to use each type of teething aid than those from non-manual backgrounds (Table 4.12). Among the children of mothers who had GCE 'A' levels and higher qualifications 13% had never used any teething aids compared with 7% among those whose mothers had 'other' (p<0.01) or no qualifications (p<0.05). Biscuits and rusks were more widely used among those whose mothers had no qualifications than among others. *(Table 4.13)*

4.5 Toothbrushing

Overall 98% of children had started having their teeth brushed or brushing their own teeth at the time of interview. *(Table 4.14)*

For just under half the children in the survey (49%) toothbrushing (by self or other) started before the age of one year and for another 40% toothbrushing started in the following year. *(Table 4.15)*

Children from non-manual backgrounds were more likely to have started having their teeth brushed or brushing their own teeth before the age of one year than those from the manual social class group (55% compared with 44%, p<0.01). *(Table 4.16)*

Table 4.12 Proportion of children who used different teething aids by social class of head of household and age of child

Social class of head of household and teething aid used	Age of child (in years)			
	$1^1/_2$ - $2^1/_2$	$2^1/_2$ - $3^1/_2$	$3^1/_2$ - $4^1/_2$	All ages
	*Percentage of children**			
Non-manual				
Balm or gel	64	66	61	64
Medicine or painkillers	71	60	57	62
Teething ring	49	44	48	47
Special biscuits/rusks	28	24	25	26
Other†	13	9	9	10
No teething aids used	9	13	14	12
Base	*226*	*268*	*246*	*740*
Manual				
Balm or gel	71	72	71	72
Medicine or painkillers	70	62	60	64
Teething ring	59	56	58	57
Special biscuits/rusks	30	29	6	6
Other†	11	9	7	9
No teething aid used	6	6	6	6
Base	*250*	*308*	*296*	*854*

* Percentages add to more than 100% as some children used more than one type of teething aid.
† Including teething granules and powders, alcohol and ice-cubes.

Table 4.13 Type of teething aids used by mother's highest educational qualification and age of child

Mother's highest educational qualification and type of teething aid used	Age of child (in years)			
	$1^1/_2$ - $2^1/_2$	$2^1/_2$ - $3^1/_2$	$3^1/_2$ - $4^1/_2$	All ages
	*Percentage of children**			
GCE 'A' level or higher				
Balm or gel	57	64	60	60
Medicine or painkillers	68	58	54	60
Teething ring	43	43	50	45
Special biscuits/rusks	24	22	26	24
Other†	13	10	9	11
No teething aids used	10	16	12	13
Base	*152*	*167*	*159*	*478*
Other				
Balm or gel	73	73	68	71
Medicine or painkillers	72	65	61	66
Teething ring	57	54	55	55
Special biscuits/rusks	26	27	29	27
Other†	11	8	6	8
No teething aids used	6	6	10	7
Base	*254*	*298*	*267*	*819*
None				
Balm or gel	71	69	73	71
Medicine or painkillers	75	55	55	60
Teething ring	62	54	60	58
Special biscuits/rusks	43	35	37	38
Other†	17	10	8	11
No teething aids used	6	11	5	7
Base	*91*	*132*	*131*	*354*

* Percentages add to more than 100% as some children used more than one type of teething aid.
† Including teething granules and powders, alcohol and ice-cubes.

Table 4.14 Whether toothbrushing started by age of child

Age of child in years	Toothbrushing started	*Base*
$1^1/_2$ - $2^1/_2$	96%	*497*
$2^1/_2$ - $3^1/_2$	98%	*598*
$3^1/_2$ - $4^1/_2$	99%	*559*
All ages	98%	*1654*

24

Table 4.15 Age when toothbrushing started by age of child

Age when toothbrushing started	Age of child (in years)			
	$1^1/_2$ - $2^1/_2$	$2^1/_2$ - $3^1/_2$	$3^1/_2$ - $4^1/_2$	All ages
	%	%	%	%
Less than 1 year	54	48	47	49
1 year - less than 2 years	41	42	38	40
2 years and over	1	9	15	9
Not yet started	4	2	1	2
Base	*497*	*598*	*559*	*1654*

4.16 Age when toothbrushing started by social class of head of household and age of child

Social class of head of household and age when toothbrushing started	Age of child (in years)			
	$1^1/_2$ - $2^1/_2$	$2^1/_2$ - $3^1/_2$	$3^1/_2$ - $4^1/_2$	All ages
	%	%	%	%
Non-manual				
Less than 1 year	55	56	54	55
1 year - less than 2 years	42	38	34	38
2 years and over	-	5	11	5
Not yet started	2	1	-	1
Base	*226*	*268*	*246*	*740*
Manual				
Less than 1 year	51	42	41	44
1 year - less than 2 years	42	44	39	42
2 years and over	2	12	18	11
Not yet started	6	2	1	3
Base	*250*	*308*	*296*	*854*

Table 4.17 Who brushes child's teeth by sex and age of child

Who brushes child's teeth	Age of child (in years)			
	$1^1/_2$ - $2^1/_2$	$2^1/_2$ - $3^1/_2$	$3^1/_2$ - $4^1/_2$	All ages
	%	%	%	%
Boys				
Child	23	32	37	31
Parent	36	23	20	26
Varies - parent or child	37	43	43	41
Brushing not started	4	3	1	3
Base	*254*	*308*	*280*	*842*
Girls				
Child	31	26	41	32
Parent	26	23	17	22
Varies - parent or child	40	51	42	45
Brushing not started	3	-	-	1
Base	*243*	*290*	*279*	*812*
Boys and girls				
Child	27	29	39	31
Parent	31	23	18	24
Varies - parent or child	38	47	42	43
Brushing not started	4	2	1	2
Base	*497*	*598*	*559*	*1654*

At the time of interview 31% of children were always brushing their own teeth (Table 4.17). Older children were more likely to have started always brushing their own teeth than younger children. Only 18% of $3^1/_2$ to $4^1/_2$ year olds always had their teeth brushed by an adult compared with 31% of those aged $1^1/_2$ to $2^1/_2$ years (p<0.01). Among each age group most children sometimes had their teeth brushed for them and sometimes brushed their own teeth. Of the 31% of children always brushing their own teeth at the time of interview, one third had always done so; this means that 10% of all children in the survey had never had their teeth brushed by an adult (table not shown).

A significantly smaller proportion of children from non-manual than from manual backgrounds always brushed their own teeth at the time of interview; 25% compared with 37% (p<0.01) (Table 4.18). Table 4.19 shows a strong relationship between mother's highest educational qualification and the person responsible for toothbrushing. Almost half the chil-

Table 4.18 Who brushes child's teeth by social class of head of household and age of child

Social class of head of household and who brushes child's teeth	Age of child (in years)			
	$1^1/_2$ - $2^1/_2$	$2^1/_2$ - $3^1/_2$	$3^1/_2$ - $4^1/_2$	All ages
	%	%	%	%
Non-manual				
Child	23	20	32	25
Parent	34	29	23	29
Varies - parent or child	42	50	45	46
Brushing not started	2	1	-	1
Base	*226*	*268*	*246*	*740*
Manual				
Child	30	36	45	37
Parent	30	18	14	20
Varies - parent or child	35	44	41	40
Brushing not started	6	2	1	3
Base	*250*	*308*	*296*	*854*

Table 4.19 Who cleans child's teeth by mother's highest educational qualification and age of child

Mother's highest educational qualification and who cleans child's teeth	Age of child (in years)			
	$1^1/_2$ - $2^1/_2$	$2^1/_2$ - $3^1/_2$	$3^1/_2$ - $4^1/_2$	All ages
	%	%	%	%
GCE 'A' level or above				
Child	19	19	25	21
Parent	38	30	30	33
Varies - parent or child	41	50	45	46
Brushing not started	1	1	-	1
Base	*152*	*167*	*159*	*478*
Other				
Child	26	30	39	32
Parent	31	21	15	22
Varies - parent or child	40	47	45	44
Brushing not started	4	1	1	2
Base	*254*	*298*	*267*	*819*
None				
Child	42	38	55	45
Parent	20	19	12	16
Varies - parent or child	30	40	33	35
Brushing not started	9	3	1	4
Base	*91*	*132*	*131*	*354*

dren whose mothers had no qualifications were always brushing their own teeth, compared with just under a third of those whose mothers had 'other' qualifications and only one in five (21%) of those whose mothers had GCE 'A' levels or a higher qualification.

Over half the children in the survey had their teeth brushed (by self or other) more than once a day (55%) and one third had their teeth brushed once a day. The remaining 12% of children had their teeth brushed less than once a day. The frequency of toothbrushing increased by age; 48% of $1^1/_2$ to $2^1/_2$ year olds had their teeth brushed more than once a day compared with 60% of those aged $3^1/_2$ to $4^1/_2$ years (p<0.01).
(Table 4.20)

Table 4.21 shows that children from the non-manual social classes were less likely than those from manual backgrounds to have their teeth brushed less than once a day (8% compared with 16%, p<0.01) and more likely to have their teeth brushed more than once a day (61% compared with 49%, p<0.01).

Table 4.20 Frequency of toothbrushing by sex and age of child

Frequency of toothbrushing	Age of child (in years)			
	$1^1/_2$ - $2^1/_2$	$2^1/_2$ - $3^1/_2$	$3^1/_2$ - $4^1/_2$	All ages
	%	%	%	%
Boys				
Less than once a day*	14	17	12	14
Once a day	39	31	32	34
More than once a day	47	52	56	52
Base	*254*	*308*	*280*	*842*
Girls				
Less than once a day*	14	8	8	10
Once a day	37	33	29	33
More than once a day	49	59	63	58
Base	*243*	*290*	*279*	*812*
Boys and girls				
Less than once a day*	14	12	10	12
Once a day	38	32	30	33
More than once a day	48	56	60	55
Base	*497*	*598*	*559*	*1654*

* Most children in this category had their teeth brushed (by self or other) at least once a week; the small number of children who had not yet started toothbrushing are also included.

Table 4.21 Frequency of toothbrushing by social class of head of household and age of child

Social class of head of household and frequency of toothbrushing	Age of child (in years)			
	$1^1/_2$ - $2^1/_2$	$2^1/_2$ - $3^1/_2$	$3^1/_2$ - $4^1/_2$	All ages
	%	%	%	%
Non-manual				
Less than once a day*	7	9	9	8
Once a day	39	29	26	31
More than once a day	54	63	66	61
Base	*226*	*268*	*246*	*740*
Manual				
Less than once a day*	20	17	12	16
Once a day	38	35	34	35
More than once a day	43	49	54	49
Base	*250*	*308*	*296*	*854*

* Most children in this category had their teeth brushed at least once a week; the small number of children who had not yet started toothbrushing are also included.

The times of day at which teeth were brushed are shown in Table 4.22. Toothbrushing took place after breakfast for over 60% of children in the survey and over 50% had their teeth brushed at bedtime, after all eating was finished for the day.

Among children whose teeth were brushed once a day, after breakfast was the most popular time for toothbrushing, followed by bedtime after all eating was finished; these accounted for 44% and 31% of cases respectively. Among children whose teeth were brushed more than once a day 79% had their teeth brushed after breakfast and 71% had their teeth brushed at bedtime after all eating was finished for the day.
(Table 4.23)

Table 4.22 Times of day when teeth brushed by age of child

Times of day when teeth brushed	Age of child (in years)			
	$1^1/_2$ - $2^1/_2$	$2^1/_2$ - $3^1/_2$	$3^1/_2$ - $4^1/_2$	All ages
	*Percentage of children * *			
Before breakfast	14	16	13	14
After breakfast	57	60	67	61
Bedtime, may eat after	21	20	15	18
Bed time, after all eating	45	51	58	52
After other meal	5	4	6	5
At other times	6	7	6	6
Varies	3	6	5	5
Teeth not brushed	4	2	1	2
Base	*497*	*598*	*559*	*1654*

* Percentages add to more than 100% as some children brushed their teeth at more than one time of day.

Table 4.23 Times of day when teeth brushed by frequency of brushing and age of child

Frequency of toothbrushing and times of day when teeth brushed	Age of child (in years)			
	$1^1/_2$ - $2^1/_2$	$2^1/_2$ - $3^1/_2$	$3^1/_2$ - $4^1/_2$	All ages
	Percentage of children			
Brushed less than once a day				
Before breakfast	8	17	9	12
After breakfast	40	31	26	32
Bedtime, may eat after	12	11	32	18
Bedtime, after eating	28	22	28	26
After other meal	8	2	-	3
At other times	6	2	6	4
Varies	10	28	15	19
Base	*50*	*64*	*53*	*167*
Brushed once a day				
Before breakfast	11	10	11	11
After breakfast	40	45	49	44
Bedtime, may eat after	16	16	7	13
Bedtime, after eating	30	30	31	31
After other meal	2	1	-	1
At other times	1	2	1	1
Varies	2	3	4	3
Base	*188*	*191*	*170*	*549*
Brushed more than once a day				
Before breakfast	19	20	14	17
After breakfast	79	76	83	79
Bedtime, may eat after	28	24	10	20
Bedtime, after eating	65	70	77	71
After other meal	8	6	10	8
At other times	10	11	8	10
Varies	3	3	4	3
Base	*239*	*331*	*333*	*903*

4.6 Fluoride use

4.6.1 Fluoride concentration of toothpaste used

The toothpastes children used were classified according to their fluoride concentration. Toothpastes formulated specifically for children with fluoride concentrations of below 600 parts per million (ppm) are referred to as low fluoride toothpastes. Medium fluoride toothpastes have fluoride concentrations of 1000 to 1100 ppm. This category includes some toothpastes which claim to be for children but which have fluoride contents within the range shown. High fluoride toothpastes are those with fluoride concentrations of approximately 1500 ppm. Where there was any doubt about the fluoride content of the toothpaste used, but it was known to fall into one of two categories, it was placed in the higher fluoride concentration category. In a few cases, toothpastes were known to contain fluoride but there was no information about the fluoride concentration; these cases are included in the category 'other'. Table 4.24 shows that low fluoride toothpastes were definitely used by 34% of children in the sample (although the true usage may be slightly higher). No more than 19% of children used high fluoride toothpastes.

Low fluoride toothpastes were used by a higher proportion of children from non-manual (43%) than manual backgrounds (27%) (p<0.01). *(Table 4.25)*

A strong association was also found between the use of low fluoride toothpastes and mothers having higher educational qualifications. *(Table 4.26)*

Table 4.27 shows the regional pattern of fluoride use. High fluoride toothpastes were more popular in Scotland than in any other area. Twenty seven per cent of Scottish children used high fluoride toothpaste compared with 20% or less in all the other regions; differences are statistically significant (p<0.05) between Scotland and the Northern region of England and Scotland and the region covering Central and South West England and Wales.

Table 4.24 Fluoride concentration of toothpaste used, by age of child

Fluoride concentration of toothpaste used	Age of child (in years)			
	$1^1/_2$ - $2^1/_2$	$2^1/_2$ - $3^1/_2$	$3^1/_2$ - $4^1/_2$	All ages
	%	%	%	%
Low fluoride	41	31	31	34
Medium fluoride	36	43	42	40
High fluoride	15	21	22	19
Other*	4	3	5	4
None	5	3	1	3
Base	*497*	*598*	*559*	*1654*

*Includes non-fluoride toothpastes (used by under 1% of children overall), toothpastes which may or may not contain fluoride and toothpastes known to contain fluoride, but in unknown concentrations.

Table 4.25 Fluoride concentration of toothpaste used, by social class of head of household and age of child

Social class of head of household and fluoride concentration of toothpaste used	Age of child (in years)			
	$1^1/_2$ - $2^1/_2$	$2^1/_2$ - $3^1/_2$	$3^1/_2$ - $4^1/_2$	All ages
	%	%	%	%
Non-manual				
Low fluoride	50	40	40	43
Medium fluoride	31	41	40	37
High fluoride	14	15	17	15
Other*	3	3	2	3
None	2	2	-	1
Base	*226*	*268*	*246*	*740*
Manual				
Low fluoride	34	23	24	27
Medium fluoride	40	45	43	43
High fluoride	15	27	25	23
Other*	4	2	6	4
None	7	4	1	4
Base	*250*	*308*	*296*	*854*

* Includes non-fluoride toothpastes (used by under 1% of children overall), toothpastes which may or may not contain fluoride and toothpastes known to contain fluoride, but in unknown concentrations.

Table 4.26 Fluoride concentration of toothpaste used, by mother's highest educational qualification and age of child

Mother's highest educational qualification and fluoride concentration of toothpaste used	Age of child (in years)			
	$1^1/_2$ - $2^1/_2$	$2^1/_2$ - $3^1/_2$	$3^1/_2$ - $4^1/_2$	All ages
	%	%	%	%
GCE 'A' level and higher				
Low fluoride	55	40	40	45
Medium fluoride	26	41	42	37
High fluoride	14	14	17	15
Other*	3	2	2	2
None	2	2	-	2
Base	*152*	*167*	*159*	*478*
Other				
Low fluoride	38	31	32	33
Medium fluoride	40	44	40	41
High fluoride	13	21	24	20
Other*	4	3	4	4
None	5	2	1	2
Base	*254*	*298*	*267*	*819*
No qualifications				
Low fluoride	26	22	20	22
Medium fluoride	39	42	47	43
High fluoride	21	29	24	25
Other*	4	3	8	5
None	10	5	2	5
Base	*91*	*132*	*131*	*354*

* Includes non-fluoride toothpastes (used by under 1% of children overall), toothpastes which may or may not contain fluoride and toothpastes known to contain fluoride, but in unknown concentrations.

Table 4.27 Fluoride concentration of toothpaste used, by region and age of child

Region and fluoride concentration of toothpaste used	Age of child (in years)			
	1½ - 2½	2½ - 3½	3½ - 4½	All ages
	%	%	%	%
Scotland				
Low fluoride	27	23	19	23
Medium fluoride	32	43	41	39
High fluoride	27	25	30	27
Other*	9	4	11	8
None	5	5	-	3
Base	*44*	*56*	*64*	*164*
North				
Low fluoride	34	34	27	32
Medium fluoride	42	39	50	44
High fluoride	16	21	16	18
Other*	2	4	6	4
None	6	2	1	3
Base	*118*	*168*	*125*	*411*
Central, South West and Wales				
Low fluoride	38	32	33	34
Medium fluoride	44	46	38	43
High fluoride	10	17	24	17
Other*	4	2	4	3
None	5	3	1	3
Base	*173*	*202*	*190*	*565*
London and South East				
Low fluoride	53	31	37	40
Medium fluoride	23	41	41	35
High fluoride	16	24	20	20
Other*	4	2	2	3
None	4	2	1	2
Base	*162*	*172*	*180*	*514*

* Includes non-fluoride toothpastes (used by under 1% of children overall), toothpastes which may or may not contain fluoride and toothpastes known to contain fluoride, but in unknown concentrations.

4.6.2 Amount of toothpaste used

Overall 92% of children were reported to use junior sized toothbrushes while 6% used adult toothbrushes (Table 4.28). In the interview the amount of toothpaste used was asked in relation to the length of the toothbrush covered by toothpaste. Table 4.29 shows the amount of toothpaste used by children of different ages. The data have been scaled where necessary to relate to a junior size toothbrush (for the 6% of children using adult toothbrushes 'small part of brush' has been scaled up to equate to 'half brush' and half an adult brush has been equated to most of a junior brush). Over 50% of children were reported to have only a small amount of toothpaste on their (junior or equivalent) brush although this measure is obviously subjective.

Table 4.30 combines brush size, toothpaste type and the amount of toothpaste used to give an indication of the amount of fluoride children use when they brush their teeth. Dentists currently recommend the use of small quantities of low fluoride toothpaste for most children. Differences were found by social class; 30% of children from non-manual backgrounds reportedly used small amounts of low fluoride toothpaste compared with 15% of those from manual backgrounds (p<0.01) (Table 4.31). Obviously the total amount

28

of fluoride children obtain from toothpaste will depend on how frequently they brush their teeth. It has already been shown that toothbrushing occurs more often among children from non-manual backgrounds than among those from households with a manual head.

Table 4.28 Size of toothbrush used by age of child

Size of toothbrush used	Age of child (in years)			
	1½ - 2½	2½ - 3½	3½ - 4½	All ages
	%	%	%	%
Junior	91	93	93	92
Adult	5	6	7	6
Not started toothbrushing	4	2	1	2
Base	*497*	*598*	*559*	*1654*

Table 4.29 Amount of toothpaste used by age of child

Amount of toothpaste used*	Age of child (in years)			
	1½ - 2½	2½ - 3½	3½ - 4½	All ages
	%	%	%	%
Covers small part of brush	58	54	46	53
Covers half length of brush	20	18	22	20
Covers most of brush	17	25	31	25
No toothpaste used	5	3	1	3
Base	*497*	*598*	*559*	*1654*

* Quantities of toothpaste scaled in relation to junior size toothbrush ('small part' of adult brush equated to 'half' a junior brush; 'half an adult brush, equated to 'most of' a junior brush).

Table 4.30 Fluoride concentration of toothpaste and amount used by age of child

Fluoride concentration of toothpaste and amount used*	Age of child (in years)			
	1½ - 2½	2½ - 3½	3½ - 4½	All ages
	%	%	%	%
Low fluoride				
covers small part of brush	28	20	18	21
covers about half of brush	7	5	7	6
covers most of brush	6	7	7	6
Medium fluoride				
covers small part of brush	20	24	17	20
covers about half of brush	9	8	10	9
covers most of brush	7	10	15	11
High fluoride				
covers small part of brush	12	12	14	13
covers about half of brush	1	1	1	1
covers most of brush	2	8	8	6
No toothpaste used or do not know fluoride content	9	5	6	7
Base	*497*	*598*	*559*	*1654*

* Quantities of toothpaste scaled in relation to junior size toothbrush ('small part' of adult brush equated to 'half' a junior brush; 'half an adult brush, equated to 'most of' a junior brush).

Table 4.31 Fluoride concentration of toothpaste and amount used by social class of head of household

Fluoride concentration of toothpaste and amount used*	Social class of head of household	
	Non-manual	Manual
	%	%
All children 1½ - 4½ years		
Low fluoride		
covers small part of brush	30	15
covers about half of brush	7	5
covers most of brush	6	7
Medium fluoride		
covers small part of brush	21	20
covers about half of brush	8	9
covers most of brush	8	13
High fluoride		
covers small part of brush	11	14
covers about half of brush	1	1
covers most of brush	4	8
No toothpaste used or do not know fluoride content	5	8
Base	*740*	*854*

* Quantities of toothpaste scaled in relation to junior size toothbrush ('small part' of adult brush equated to 'half' a junior brush; 'half an adult brush, equated to 'most of' a junior brush).

4.6.3 Use of fluoride supplements [1]

Eighteen per cent of children had taken fluoride supplements in tablet or drop form (Table 4.32). A higher proportion of children from non-manual than from manual backgrounds had taken fluoride supplements (22% compared with 14%, p<0.01).   *(Table 4.33)*

The use of fluoride supplements varied significantly by region; over half the children in Scotland were using or had used fluoride supplements compared with less than a quarter of those in London and the South East and only about one in ten of those in the North and Central and South West England and Wales (p<0.01).   *(Table 4.34)*

The age at which children started taking fluoride supplements is shown in Table 4.35; of the children taking fluoride supplements, most began before the age of one year.

Although 97% of children taking fluoride supplements were also using fluoride toothpaste (table not shown), no pattern was identified between the use of fluoride supplements and the fluoride concentration or amount of toothpaste used.

Table 4.32 Use of fluoride supplements by age of child

Use of fluoride supplements	Age of child (in years)			
	1½ - 2½	2½ - 3½	3½ - 4½	All ages
	%	%	%	%
Used now	7	5	7	6
Used in past	9	13	13	12
Never used	84	82	80	82
Base	*497*	*598*	*559*	*1654*

Table 4.33 Use of fluoride supplements by social class of head of household and age of child

Social class of head of household and use of fluoride supplements	Age of child (in years)			
	1½ - 2½	2½ - 3½	3½ - 4½	All ages
	%	%	%	%
Non-manual				
Used now	8	6	9	8
Used in past	10	15	17	14
Never used	82	79	74	78
Base	*226*	*268*	*246*	*740*
Manual				
Used now	6	4	5	5
Used in past	8	11	9	9
Never used	86	85	86	86
Base	*250*	*308*	*296*	*854*

Table 4.34 Use of fluoride supplements by region and age of child

Region and use of fluoride supplements	Age of child (in years)			
	1½ - 2½	2½ - 3½	3½ - 4½	All ages
	%	%	%	%
Scotland				
Used now	23	11	22	18
Used in past	34	36	28	32
Never used	43	54	50	49
Base	*44*	*56*	*64*	*164*
Northern				
Used now	6	7	6	6
Used in past	4	5	6	5
Never used	90	88	87	88
Base	*118*	*168*	*125*	*411*
Central, South West and Wales				
Used now	5	2	2	3
Used in past	6	9	5	7
Never used	89	89	93	90
Base	*173*	*202*	*190*	*565*
London and South East				
Used now	6	5	8	6
Used in past	9	18	21	16
Never used	85	77	71	78
Base	*162*	*172*	*180*	*514*

Table 4.35 Age when child started using fluoride supplements by age of child

Age started using fluoride supplements	Age of child (in years)			
	1½ - 2½	2½ - 3½	3½ - 4½	All ages
	%	%	%	%
Under 6 months	5	4	3	4
6 months - less than 1 year	7	8	7	7
1 year - less than 2 years	4	4	4	4
2 years or over	-	2	6	3
Never used	84	82	80	82
Base	*497*	*598*	*559*	*1654*

4.6.4 Use of fluoride supplements and fluoride advice

Table 4.36 shows whether children were taking fluoride supplements and the advice their parents had received about fluoride. Two thirds of parents who had been advised to give their child fluoride had done so; 26% were doing so at the time of interview. Of those who had been advised not to give their child fluoride supplements, 29% had done so at some time, although only 8% were giving them at the time of interview. Some of these parents had also received advice to give their child fluoride supplements; overall 4% of parents had received advice both to give, and not to give, their child fluoride supplements (table not shown). Of those who had received no advice at all about fluoride, 96% had never given their child supplements.

4.7 Mother's dental attendance pattern and child's visits to a dentist

The attitude of parents towards their child's dental care may reflect their own dental experience. Table 4.37 shows that 60% of mothers classified themselves as regular attenders at

the dentist and 13% considered themselves to be occasional attenders, while 25% only went to the dentist when they were having trouble with their teeth. This pattern is identical to that found for women aged 25 to 34 years in the 1988 Adult dental health survey[3] (Table not shown).

Table 4.38 compares the dental experience of children with their mothers' dental attendance patterns and shows that the children of regular attenders were far more likely to have been seen and examined by a dentist (63%) than children whose mothers went to the dentist occasionally (37%) or when they had trouble with their teeth (33%) (p<0.01).

Table 4.36 Use of fluoride supplements by whether parents received advice to give child fluoride and age of child

Fluoride advice and use of supplements	Age of child (in years)			
	$1^1/_2$ - $2^1/_2$	$2^1/_2$ - $3^1/_2$	$3^1/_2$ - $4^1/_2$	All ages
	%	%	%	%
Advised to give child fluoride				
Child using supplements	31	20	27	26
Child used supplements in past	31	48	45	42
Never used	37	32	28	32
Base	*105*	*133*	*135*	*373*
Advised not to give child fluoride				
Child using supplements	13	7	4	8
Child used supplements in past	13	24	24	21
Never used	73	70	72	71
Base	*45*	*59*	*50*	*154*
No fluoride advice				
Child using supplements	1	1	1	1
Child used supplements in past	3	3	3	3
Never used	96	97	96	96
Base	*365*	*430*	*395*	*1190*

Table 4.37 Mother's dental attendance pattern by age of child

Mother's dental attendance pattern	Age of child (in years)			
	$1^1/_2$ - $2^1/_2$	$2^1/_2$ - $3^1/_2$	$3^1/_2$ - $4^1/_2$	All ages
	%	%	%	%
Visits regularly	57	60	62	60
Visits occasionally	16	12	12	13
Visits only with trouble	24	26	23	25
Don't know	3	2	2	2
Base	*497*	*598*	*559*	*1654*

Table 4.38 Child's visits to the dentist by mother's dental attendance pattern and age of child

Mother's dental attendance pattern and child's visits to the dentist	Age of child (in years)			
	$1^1/_2$ - $2^1/_2$	$2^1/_2$ - $3^1/_2$	$3^1/_2$ - $4^1/_2$	All ages
	%	%	%	%
Mother visits regularly				
Child seen and examined	35	61	88	63
Child seen, not examined	12	12	4	9
Child never seen by dentist	53	27	8	27
Base	*285*	*356*	*347*	*988*
Mother visits occasionally				
Child seen and examined	10	48	55	37
Child seen, not examined	10	4	10	8
Child never seen by dentist	80	48	35	55
Base	*80*	*73*	*69*	*222*
Mother visits only with trouble				
Child seen and examined	9	30	57	33
Child seen, not examined	1	3	2	2
Child never seen by dentist	90	67	42	65
Base	*119*	*158*	*131*	*408*

Notes and references

[1] Fluoride supplements are not nutritional supplements. The terminology is used in this Report to reflect common usage in the dental profession.

[2] The categories listed in Table 4.10 are as they appeared in the questionnaire. Respondents were asked whether their child had used each type of teething aid separately, with no need to choose between items. Some 'balms' and 'gels' on the market are in fact medicines, however it is not known how many respondents were aware of this and so included such products in 'medicines or painkillers' as well as 'balms or gels'.On the questionnaire some respondents named gripe water, Anbesol, milk of magnesia and calpol, under 'anything else'. These have all been included with 'medicine or painkillers'. Alcohol appeared separately on the questionnaire but due to the small number of cases where this applied, it has been included in the category 'other'.

[3] Todd J E Lader D. *Adult dental health 1988, United Kingdom.* HMSO (1991).

(The Adult dental health report used specific criteria to classify people as regular or occasional dental attenders, or those who visited the dentist only when having trouble with their teeth. In this survey mothers were simply asked to classify themselves in one of these categories).

5 The use of bottles, dinky feeders and dummies and the consumption of foods and drinks containing sugars

5.1 Introduction

This chapter is concerned with drinking and eating practices thought to be related to dental decay. Information was collected during the dental interview about children's use of bottles, dinky feeders[1] and dummies and about drinks consumed at night. In addition, data relating to the consumption of confectionery and foods containing sugars from the dietary survey interview and 4-day weighed intake diary, are reported on. Household expenditure on sweets and chocolates, recorded in the dental interview is also presented.

5.2 The use of bottles

In the dental interview parents were asked whether their child had ever used a bottle. Information was collected on the age at which children started and, for those not currently using a bottle, the age when they stopped. Information was also collected about how often a bottle was used and the drinks it contained during the day and at night.

Parents were not asked about changes in their child's use of bottles over time. For children using bottles at the time of interview, questions were asked about their current practices, while the parents of children no longer using bottles were asked questions relating to the period immediately before their child stopped usage. The following analyses focus on children who were using bottles at the time of interview; some information relating to children's past use of bottles is included in Appendix C.[2]

Eighty seven per cent of children in the survey had used bottles at some time. Although no significant differences were found by age or sex, a higher proportion of children from manual (92%) than from non-manual backgrounds (83%) were reported ever to have used bottles (p<0.01). Half of those aged $1^1/_2$ to $2^1/_2$ years (49%) and 8% of those aged $3^1/_2$ to $4^1/_2$ years, were reported to be current bottle users.

(Tables 5.1 and 5.2)

Table 5.3 shows the age at which children started and stopped using bottles. Almost all children who used bottles (91%) started before the age of 6 months. The data for $3^1/_2$ to $4^1/_2$ year olds give the best indication of the age at which children stopped using bottles; most children can be seen to have

Table 5.1 Whether children had ever used, or currently used bottles, by age

Use of bottles	Age of child (in years)			
	$1^1/_2$ - $2^1/_2$	$2^1/_2$ - $3^1/_2$	$3^1/_2$ - $4^1/_2$	All ages
	%	%	%	%
Using at time of interview	49	24	8	26
Used in the past	40 89	63 87	79 87	61 87
Never used	11	13	13	13
Base	497	598	559	1654

Table 5.2 Whether children had ever used, or currently used bottles, by age and social class of head of household

Social class of head of household and use of bottles	Age of child (in years)			
	$1^1/_2$ - $2^1/_2$	$2^1/_2$ - $3^1/_2$	$3^1/_2$ - $4^1/_2$	All ages
	%	%	%	%
Non-manual				
Using at time of interview	45	26	8	26
Used in the past	40 85	56 83	73 81	57 83
Never used	15	17	20	17
Base	226	268	246	740
Manual				
Using at time of interview	52	23	9	27
Used in past	40 92	68 91	83 92	65 92
Never used	8	9	8	8
Base	250	308	296	854

Table 5.3 Age when bottle users started and stopped use by age

Age when started and stopped using bottle	Age of child (in years)			
	$1^1/_2$ - $2^1/_2$	$2^1/_2$ - $3^1/_2$	$3^1/_2$ - $4^1/_2$	All ages
	%	%	%	%
Age started use				
Less than 6 months	92	90	90	91
6 months - less than 1 year	6	9	8	8
1 year and over	2	1	1	2
Age stopped use				
Less than 6 months	2	1	1	1
6 months - less than 1 year	15	20	19	18
1 year - less than 2 years	24	38	44	36
2 years - less than 3 years	4	11	19	12
Over 3 years	-	1	7	3
Still using	55	28	10	30
Base	440	521	485	1446

stopped by the age of 2 years. The patterns of starting and stopping bottle use did not vary significantly for children from manual and non-manual social class backgrounds.

Younger children used bottles more frequently during the day than older children. For example, at the time of interview, 12% of all $1^1/_2$ to $2^1/_2$ year olds were having a bottle four or more times a day, compared with 5% of those aged $2^1/_2$ to $3^1/_2$ years and 1% of those aged $3^1/_2$ to $4^1/_2$ years (p<0.01). Among $3^1/_2$ to $4^1/_2$ year olds only 6% of children were reported ever to use bottles during the day compared with 40% of those in the youngest age cohort (p<0.01).

(Table 5.4)

Bottle use at night was also more frequent among younger children than older children. Thirty one per cent of $1^1/_2$ to $2^1/_2$ year olds were using bottles every night and a further 4% were using them some nights. Six per cent of $3^1/_2$ to $4^1/_2$ year olds were reported to use a bottle in bed every night.

(Table 5.5)

Table 5.4 Whether children currently use bottles during the day and the frequency of use, by age

Use of bottles during the day	Age of child (in years)			
	1½ - 2½	2½ - 3½	3½ - 4½	All ages
	%	%	%	%
Use 4 times or more a day	12	5	1	6
Use 3 times a day	5	3	1	3
Use twice a day	10 [40]	4 [19]	2 [6]	5 [21]
Use once a day	11	4	2	5
Use less than once a day	3	3	1	2
Never currently use during the day	60	81	94	79
Base	*497*	*598*	*559*	*1654*

Table 5.5 Whether children currently use bottles at night and the frequency of use, by age

Use of bottles at night	Age of child (in years)			
	1½ - 2½	2½ - 3½	3½ - 4½	All ages
	%	%	%	%
Use every night	31 [35]	15 [19]	6 [6]	17 [20]
Use some nights	4	4	1	3
Never currently use at night	65	81	94	80
Base	*497*	*598*	*559*	*1654*

In the dental interview over 20 types of drinks were separately identified, however for the purpose of analysis, these have been grouped into four categories as follows:

milk	cow's milk, infant formula, breast milk
water	water
drinks containing non-milk extrinsic (NME) sugars	fruit squash with sugar, hot chocolate, Ovaltine, Horlicks, flavoured milk, tea and coffee with sugar, blackcurrant drink, fruit juice or syrup, carbonated drinks (including low calorie carbonated drinks)[3]
other drinks, not containing NME sugars	fruit squash without sugar, low calorie blackcurrant drink, tea or coffee without sugar

Non-milk extrinsic sugars[4] are considered to be particularly likely to contribute to dental caries; milk contains milk-sugars, however these are less damaging to the teeth.[5]

Over half the children using bottles at night usually had milk in them (56%) while a quarter (24%) usually had a drink containing NME sugars (Table 5.6). Among 3½ to 4½ year olds still taking a bottle to bed at night, 42% had a drink containing NME sugars, and the consumption of milk from bottles was correspondingly lower than among the younger children. Children from manual and non-manual social class backgrounds were found not to take different types of drinks to bed in their bottles.

Table 5.6 Usual drinks consumed from bottles during the night, among children using bottles at night at the time of interview, by age

Drinks consumed from bottles during the night	Age of child (in years)			
	1½ - 2½	2½ - 3½	3½ - 4½	All ages
	%	%	%	%
Milk	56	60	42	56
Drink containing, NME sugars	24	20	42	24
Water	5	7	3	6
Other drink, not containing NME sugars	14	13	14	14
Base	*174*	*114*	*36*	*324*

5.3 The use of dinky feeders

Information similar to that collected on the use of bottles was collected in relation to dinky feeders. Eighteen per cent of children in the sample had ever used a dinky feeder; 2% were using one at the time of interview. *(Table 5.7)*

Just over half (54%) of dinky feeder users started usage before the age of 6 months; a further 36% started use between the ages of 6 months and one year. Dinky feeder users tended to stop use earlier than bottle users; almost a fifth of users (19%) had stopped using a dinky feeder before the age of 6 months (Table 5.8).

Only 3% of children in the survey ever took a dinky feeder to bed. At the time of interview, 1% of children were using a dinky feeder once or twice a day and 1% were using dinky feeders more than twice a day (Tables not shown).

Table 5.7 Whether children had ever used, or currently used dinky feeders, by age

Use of dinky feeders	Age of child (in years)			
	1½ - 2½	2½ - 3½	3½ - 4½	All ages
	%	%	%	%
Using at time of interview	3 [17]	2 [18]	1 [18]	2 [18]
Used in the past	14	17	18	16
Never used	83	82	82	82
Base	*497*	*598*	*559*	*1654*

Table 5.8 Age when dinky feeder users started and stopped use by age

Age when started and stopped using dinky feeders	Age of child (in years)			
	1½ - 2½	2½ - 3½	3½ - 4½	All ages
	%	%	%	%
Age started use				
Less than 6 months	69	53	44	54
6 months - less than 1 year	23	37	46	36
1 year and over	8	9	10	9
Age stopped use				
Less than 6 months	29	18	12	19
6 months - less than 1 year	22	19	26	22
1 year - less than 2 years	31	40	34	35
2 years - less than 3 years	1	14	21	13
Over 3 years	-	-	4	1
Still using	17	8	3	9
Base	*84*	*110*	*103*	*297*

Of all those who had ever used a dinky feeder, 94% had used one during the day. The usual drinks consumed from dinky-feeders during the day are shown in Table 5.9; the information for current and past users has been combined because of the low prevalence of current dinky feeder use. Although not ideal, this does show that drinks containing NME sugars[4] were more commonly consumed from dinky feeders than were other drinks.

5.4 The use of dummies

Just over half the children in the survey (53%) had ever used a dummy. At the time of interview, 39% of those aged $1^1/_2$ to $2^1/_2$ years and 10% of $3^1/_2$ to $4^1/_2$ year olds were using dummies. *(Table 5.10)*

A higher proportion of children from manual than from non-manual backgrounds were reported to have used dummies (62% compared with 43%, p<0.01, table not shown).

Parents were asked whether their child's dummy had ever been dipped into anything sweet to make it taste nice; 5% of children had been given a sweetened dummy (table not shown).

Most children (95%) who ever used a dummy started before the age of six months; 10% also stopped before the age of six months (Table 5.11). Looking at the ages when children in the $3^1/_2$ to $4^1/_2$ age cohort stopped using dummies, it can be seen that about a quarter of users (23%) stopped between the ages of one and two years, followed by a further quarter (26%) stopping before the age of three years. A fifth (19%) had not stopped usage at the time of interview.

All current dummy users were reported to use their dummies in bed.

Table 5.9 The drinks which children who were using dinky feeders at the time of interview, or who had used them in the past, were reported to consume from them most frequently during the day

Drinks consumed from dinky feeders during the day	Children aged $1^1/_2$ to $4^1/_2$ years
	%
Milk	11
Drink containing NME sugars	39
Water	11
Other drink, not containing NME sugars	22
Don't know	11
Never used dinky feeder during the day	6
Base	*297*

Table 5.10 Whether children had ever used, or currently used dummies, by age

Use of dummies	Age of child (in years)			
	$1^1/_2$ - $2^1/_2$	$2^1/_2$ - $3^1/_2$	$3^1/_2$ - $4^1/_2$	All ages
	%	%	%	%
Using at time of interview	39	22	10	23
Used in the past	17 (56)	29 (51)	43 (53)	30 (53)
Never used	44	49	47	47
Base	*497*	*598*	*559*	*1654*

Table 5.11 Age when dummy users started and stopped use by age

Age when started and stopped using dummy	Age of child (in years)			
	$1^1/_2$ - $2^1/_2$	$2^1/_2$ - $3^1/_2$	$3^1/_2$ - $4^1/_2$	All ages
	%	%	%	%
Age started use				
Less than 6 months	96	97	93	95
6 months - less than 1 year	3	2	4	3
1 year and over	1	1	2	1
Age stopped use				
Less than 6 months	11	6	12	10
6 months - less than 1 year	7	10	7	8
1 year - less than 2 years	11	19	23	18
2 years - less than 3 years	2	19	26	16
Over 3 years	-	3	12	5
Still using	70	43	19	43
Base	*277*	*307*	*298*	*882*

5.5 Drinks in bed and during the night

In addition to the detailed information collected about children's use of bottles and dinky feeders, data were also obtained about drinks consumed by children in bed and during the night. Just under a third (31%) of children were reported to have a drink in bed every night and almost half of those in the survey (48%) sometimes, or always had a drink in bed. *(Table 5.12)*

Table 5.13 shows the drinks children consumed in bed (for those who did not always have the same drink, the drink consumed most frequently was recorded); those having a drink every night are shown separately from those having a night-time drink less frequently. Milk was drunk most often by 24% of $1^1/_2$ to $2^1/_2$ year olds and by 9% of those aged $3^1/_2$ to $4^1/_2$ years. Compared with other drinks, milk was the most popular drink for all children having a drink every night and the least popular drink among those having a drink some nights; water was the most popular drink among those having a drink some nights. In each age cohort, 12% of children had a drink containing non-milk extrinsic sugars in bed; two thirds of these children had a drink every night (see section 5.2 for an explanation of how drinks were classified).

Children aged $1^1/_2$ to $2^1/_2$ were most likely to drink from a bottle at night while those aged $3^1/_2$ to $4^1/_2$ years were most likely to drink from a mug, cup or glass (Table 5.14). Overall children drinking in bed every night were more likely to use a bottle than any other vessel while those who had a drink some nights were most likely to use a mug, cup or glass. These differences are largely due to those having a drink every night including a higher proportion of younger than older children, while older children dominated the group who had a drink some nights.

For each type of drinking vessel the types of drinks consumed at night are shown in Table 5.15. Milk was the most popular drink consumed from a bottle, being the usual drink for over half the children (54%) using a bottle at night. Only 6% of bottle users usually drank water at night. Among children using feeder beakers,[6] the proportions drinking milk (27%), water (23%) and drinks containing NME sugars (30%) and other drinks not containing NME sugars (20%) were of a similar order. Water was the most commonly consumed drink from mugs, cups and glasses, with 39% of users usually drinking water at night.

Table 5.12 Whether children were reported to have a drink in bed at the time of interview and the frequency of having drinks in bed, by age

Frequency of having a drink in bed	Age of child (in years)			
	$1^1/_2$ - $2^1/_2$	$2^1/_2$ - $3^1/_2$	$3^1/_2$ - $4^1/_2$	All ages
	%	%	%	%
Have drink in bed:				
Every night	39	32	22	31
1 to 6 nights a week	7　51	10　48	13　44	10　48
Less than once a week	5	6	9	7
Never have drink in bed	49	52	56	52
Base	*497*	*598*	*559*	*1654*

Table 5.13 How often children were reported to have a drink in bed at the time of interview, and the usual drinks taken to bed, by age

How often have drink in bed and type of drink taken to bed	Age of child (in years)			
	$1^1/_2$ - $2^1/_2$	$2^1/_2$ - $3^1/_2$	$3^1/_2$ - $4^1/_2$	All ages
	%	%	%	%
Never have drink in bed	49	52	56	52
Have drink in bed every night:				
Milk	21	13	6	13
Drink containing NME sugars	9	8	7	8
Water	4	4	4	4
Other drink, not containing NME sugars	5	6	5	6
Have drink in bed some nights:				
Milk	3	4	3	3
Drink containing NME sugars	3	4	5	4
Water	3	5	10	6
Other drink, not containing NME sugars	2	3	4	3
Base	*497*	*598*	*559*	*1654*

Table 5.14 How often children were reported to have a drink in bed at the time of interview, and the drinking vessels they usually used, by age

How often have drink in bed and drinking vessel usually used	Age of child (in years)			
	$1^1/_2$ - $2^1/_2$	$2^1/_2$ - $3^1/_2$	$3^1/_2$ - $4^1/_2$	All ages
	%	%	%	%
Never have drink in bed	49	52	56	52
Have drink in bed every night, usually in a:				
Bottle	30	14	6	16
Beaker	7	10	6	8
Mug, cup or glass	1	7	10	6
Have drink in bed some nights, usually in a:				
Bottle	3	3	1	2
Beaker	6	6	4	5
Mug, cup or glass	2	7	18	10
Base	*497*	*598*	*559*	*1654*

Table 5.15 Drinks children were reported to consume from different vessels most often in bed at the time of interview, by age

Vessels usually used in bed and the drinks most often consumed from them	Age of child (in years)			
	$1^1/_2$ - $2^1/_2$	$2^1/_2$ - $3^1/_2$	$3^1/_2$ - $4^1/_2$	All ages
	%	%	%	%
Bottle:				
Milk	55	56	41	54
Water	6	9	3	6
Drink containing NME sugars	24	18	41	24
Other drink, not containing NME sugars	15	16	15	15
Base	*161*	*101*	*34*	*296*
Feeder-beaker:				
Milk	31	26	23	27
Water	25	22	21	23
Drink containing NME sugars	25	31	34	30
Other drink, not containing NME sugars	17	21	23	20
Base	*64*	*94*	*53*	*211*
Mug, cup or glass:				
Milk	[4]	17	16	17
Water	[10]	33	41	39
Drink containing NME sugars	[3]	26	22	23
Other drink, not containing NME sugars	[1]	23	20	20
Base	*17*	*86*	*157*	*260*

Children from non-manual social class backgrounds were more likely than those from households with a manual head to have a drink in bed. The difference was especially marked among older children; among $3^1/_2$ to $4^1/_2$ year olds, 52% of children from non-manual backgrounds had a drink in bed, compared with 38% of those from manual backgrounds (p<0.01). There were some apparent differences in the types of drink consumed at night by children from manual and non-manual households; for example, among those who consumed drinks at night, 28% of $1^1/_2$ to $2^1/_2$ year olds from households with a manual head had drinks containing, NME sugars, compared with 18% of those of the same age from non-manual backgrounds. However, these differences did not reach statistical significance (p>0.05).

(Tables 5.16 and 5.17)

Table 5.16 Whether children were reported to have a drink in bed at the time of interview and the frequency of having drinks in bed, by social class of the head of household and age

Social class of head of household and frequency of having a drink in bed	Age of child (in years)			
	$1^1/_2$ - $2^1/_2$	$2^1/_2$ - $3^1/_2$	$3^1/_2$ - $4^1/_2$	All ages
	%	%	%	%
Non-manual				
Every night	36	37	25	33
1 to 6 nights a week	8	10	16	12
Less than once a week	3	9	11	8
Never	52	44	47	48
Base	*226*	*268*	*246*	*740*
Manual				
Every night	41	28	20	29
1 to 6 nights a week	6	10	11	9
Less than once a week	6	5	7	6
Never	48	58	63	56
Base	*250*	*308*	*296*	*854*

Table 5.17 Types of drink consumed in bed or during the night among children who had drinks in bed, by social class of head of household and age

Social class of head of household and types of drink had in bed	Age of child (in years)			
	1^1/$_2$ - 2^1/$_2$	2^1/$_2$ - 3^1/$_2$	3^1/$_2$ - 4^1/$_2$	All ages
	%	%	%	%
Non-manual				
Milk	51	39	21	36
Water	18	19	34	24
Drink containing NME sugars	18	24	25	23
Other drink, not containing NME sugars	13	18	20	17
Base	*108*	*150*	*129*	*387*
Manual				
Milk	45	30	20	32
Water	10	22	27	20
Drink containing NME sugars	28	25	32	28
Other drink, not containing NME sugars	17	23	22	20
Base	*131*	*131*	*111*	*373*

5.6 Eating at night

Five per cent of children in the survey were reported ever to have something to eat in bed or during the night; 1% had something to eat in bed every night (Table 5.18). Parents were asked what their children usually ate in bed (up to four answers could be given); 2% of children consumed sweet biscuits and 1% consumed each of savoury biscuits, crisps and savoury snacks and savoury sandwiches; other foods were consumed by less than 1% of children in the survey.

(Table 5.19)

Table 5.18 Whether children were reported to have food in bed at the time of interview and the frequency with which they had food at night, by age

Consumption of food at night	Age of child (in years)			
	1^1/$_2$ - 2^1/$_2$	2^1/$_2$ - 3^1/$_2$	3^1/$_2$ - 4^1/$_2$	All ages
	%	%	%	%
Had food in bed:				
Every night	-	1	2	1
4 to 6 nights a week	0	0	1	1
1 to 3 nights a week	1 (2)	1 (4)	1 (8)	1 (5)
Less than once a week	1	3	4	2
Never had food in bed	98	96	92	95
Base	*497*	*598*	*559*	*1654*

Table 5.19 Types of food consumed in bed or during the night, by age

Types of food consumed in bed	Age of child (in years)			
	1^1/$_2$ - 2^1/$_2$	2^1/$_2$ - 3^1/$_2$	3^1/$_2$ - 4^1/$_2$	All ages
	Percentage of children *			
Sweet biscuits	1	2	3	2
Savoury biscuits	0	1	2	1
Crisps or savoury snacks	0	1	1	1
Savoury sandwiches	-	1	2	1
Sweets or chocolate	0	0	1	0
Sweet sandwiches	-	1	1	0
Fruit	-	0	1	0
No food consumed in bed	98	96	92	95
Base	*497*	*598*	*559*	*1654*

* Percentages may add to more than 100% as some children consumed more than one type of food in bed.

5.7 Consumption of foods containing sugars

There is a large body of evidence relating dental caries to the consumption of sugars.[7] In linking this dental health survey to the dietary survey, it was hoped to investigate the relationship between the consumption of foods containing sugars and dental decay.

5.7.1 Data from the dietary interview (food frequency questions)

The main source of information about children's diets from the dietary survey is the four-day weighed intake diary. However there are some foods that children may eat relatively infrequently which may not appear in the four-day diary. To obtain a wider view of children's diets, the dietary interview included questions about the frequency with which children were said to eat certain foods including breakfast cereals, cakes, cheese, eggs and liver (the food frequency grid showing the full list of foods is on pages 14 and 15 of the dietary survey questionnaire in Appendix B). These data are also available for children without complete diary records. Some of the foods included on the food frequency questionnaire were high in sugars and frequent consumption of these foods might be expected to be related to experience of dental decay. The proportion of children reported to consume selected foods containing sugars with different frequencies is shown in Tables 5.20 to 5.22 (each table considers a different age cohort). In each age cohort 21% of children reportedly ate biscuits more than once a day and a further 20% to 24% had biscuits once a day. Sugar confectionery was eaten more than once a day by 3% of 1^1/$_2$ to 2^1/$_2$ year olds, 5% of 2^1/$_2$ to 3^1/$_2$ year olds and 4% of 3^1/$_2$ to 4^1/$_2$ year olds. 'Blackcurrant drinks' were consumed more than once a day by between 14% and 16% of children, and carbonated drinks (including diet carbonated drinks but excluding water[3]) were consumed more than once a day by 3% of those aged 1^1/$_2$ to 2^1/$_2$ years and 8% and 9% of those aged 2^1/$_2$ to 3^1/$_2$ years and 3^1/$_2$ to 4^1/$_2$ years respectively.

The relationships between the frequency of consumption of different foods containing sugars and dental decay are shown in the following chapter. For many of the foods listed strong relationships with dental decay in the sample were not found. The consumption of sugar confectionery and carbonated drinks were associated with dental decay, and consumption patterns by social class for these foods are shown in Table 5.23. Overall 43% of children had sugar confectionery most days or more often and 24% had carbonated drinks on at least most days; the proportions consuming both with this frequency, increased with age. Children from manual backgrounds were more likely to consume sugar confectionery and carbonated drinks most days of the week, or more often, than were those from non-manual backgrounds. For example, 41% of 1^1/$_2$ to 2^1/$_2$ year olds from manual backgrounds ate sugar confectionery with this frequency, and the proportion rose to 56% among those aged 2^1/$_2$ to 3^1/$_2$ years. Among children from non-manual backgrounds, by the age of 3^1/$_2$ to 4^1/$_2$ years only 39% of children were found to be eating sugar confectionery on most days of the week.

5.7.2 Data from the four-day weighed intake diary

The parents of 95% of children in the dental survey completed the four-day weighed intake dietary record; this

Table 5.20 Frequency with which children aged 1½ to 2½ years were reported to consume various foods containing sugars

Food frequency data

Type of food		Children aged 1½ to 2½ years*						
		Frequency of consumption						
		More than once a day	Once a day	Most days	At least once a week	At least once a month	Less than once a month	Never
Sugar confectionery	%	3	11	20	35	9	8	16
Chocolate confectionery	%	2	13	19	51	9	2	5
Biscuits - any	%	21	24	37	14	2	1	1
Cakes	%	0	4	8	53	20	10	5
Ice cream or ice lollies	%	1	5	8	32	23	17	13
Carbonated drinks†	%	3	4	9	22	10	9	42
Blackcurrant drinks	%	14	5	10	10	9	9	44
Fruit juice	%	12	9	14	18	12	7	28

* Base = 497 (Row percentages total 100%).
† Including diet carbonated drinks, but excluding mineral water.

Table 5.21 Frequency with which children aged 2½ to 3½ years were reported to consume various foods containing sugars

Food frequency data

Type of food		Children aged 2½ to 3½ years*						
		Frequency of consumption						
		More than once a day	Once a day	Most days	At least once a week	At least once a month	Less than once a month	Never
Sugar confectionery	%	5	15	27	33	9	4	8
Chocolate confectionery	%	5	13	24	46	7	4	2
Biscuits - any	%	21	21	38	17	2	1	0
Cakes	%	1	6	8	56	19	7	3
Ice cream or ice lollies	%	1	7	11	39	22	11	9
Carbonated drinks†	%	8	6	13	30	13	10	20
Blackcurrant drinks	%	14	5	11	11	11	8	42
Fruit juice	%	11	10	14	20	10	8	27

* Base = 601 (Row percentages total 100%).
† Including diet carbonated drinks, but excluding mineral water.

Table 5.22 Frequency with which children aged 3½ to 4½ years were reported to consume various foods containing sugars

Food frequency data

Type of food		Children aged 3½ to 4½ years *						
		Frequency of consumption						
		More than once a day	Once a day	Most days	At least once a week	At least a month	Less than a month	Never
Sugar confectionery	%	4	16	28	41	6	3	3
Chocolate confectionery	%	4	13	21	48	9	3	1
Biscuits - any	%	21	20	39	17	2	0	0
Cakes	%	1	4	10	56	18	6	5
Ice cream or ice lollies	%	1	5	14	41	22	13	5
Carbonated drinks †	%	9	9	12	30	12	11	17
Blackcurrant drinks	%	16	6	11	13	13	9	33
Fruit juice	%	9	9	13	23	13	8	25

* Base = 560 (Row percentages total 100%).
† Including diet carbonated drinks, but excluding mineral water.

Table 5.23 Proportion of children who were reported to consume sugar confectionery and carbonated drinks* on at least most days of the week, by social class of head of household and age

Food frequency data

Type of food consumed on at least most days of the week and social class of head of household	Age of child (in years)			
	$1^1/_2 - 2^1/_2$	$2^1/_2 - 3^1/_2$	$3^1/_2 - 4^1/_2$	All ages
	%	%	%	%
Sugar confectionery				
Non-manual	24	36	39	33
Manual	41	56	52	50
All	33	47	47	43
Carbonated drinks *				
Non-manual	9	15	19	15
Manual	22	35	37	32
All	16	26	29	24
Bases				
Non-manual	*226*	*269*	*246*	*741*
Manual	*250*	*309*	*296*	*855*
All	*497*	*601*	*560*	*1658*

* Including diet carbonated drinks, but excluding mineral water.

provides additional data about the consumption of foods containing sugars and about intakes of selected nutrients. Parents were asked to record over two week days and both weekend days, the exact type and weight of food and drink their child consumed, at the time of consumption, in a diary.[8] From the food descriptions, codes from the MAFF nutrient database[9] were assigned to each food, enabling the amounts of each separate nutrient in the foods consumed to be calculated. Data for the four day recording period were weighted[10] to give weekly consumption values for different types of food, and for 54 nutrients including carbohydrate, protein, fat, fatty acids, sugars, vitamins and minerals. These weekly data were then divided by seven to produce values for the average daily intake of nutrients. More information about the dietary data is contained in the report of the NDNS diet and nutrition survey.[11]

Many foods contain sugars in different quantities and in different forms. Certain food groups were identified which included foods containing sugars that might be damaging to children's teeth. These food groups are listed as a footnote to Tables 5.24 and 5.25; in this Report, foods from these selected food groups are collectively referred to as 'sugary foods'. It should be noted that not all of the foods in the group are necessarily high sugar foods (for example, some yogurts). Measures were derived from the weighed intake data which were intended to show the frequency of consumption of sugary foods, the quantity consumed (in grams) of these foods and also the total intake (in grams) of certain nutrients from all foods. In addition, particular interest was focused on the frequency of consumption and average daily intakes (in grams) of sugar confectionery and chocolate confectionery, soft drinks (fruit squashes with sugar and carbonated drinks) and fruit juices. Table 5.24 shows the mean and median intakes of these sugary foods and drinks and selected nutrients, for children in each age cohort. These values are compared for children with and without experience of caries in Chapter 6 of this Report. Chapter 6 also looks at children who were high and low consumers of certain sugary foods and the selected nutrients to see whether they had significantly different levels of dental decay. Table 5.25 shows consumption values at the tenth and ninetieth percentiles.

Table 5.24 Average daily frequency of consumption of selected foods containing sugars and average daily intake of these foods and selected nutrients, by age

Weighed intake data

Average daily frequency of consumption of sugary foods and average daily intake of these foods and selected nutrients	Age of child (in years)					
	$1^1/_2 - 2^1/_2$		$2^1/_2 - 3^1/_2$		$3^1/_2 - 4^1/_2$	
	Mean	Median*	Mean	Median*	Mean	Median*
Average daily frequency of consumption of:						
Sugar confectionery	0.2	0	0.4	0.1	0.4	0.4
Chocolate confectionery	0.4	0.4	0.5	0.4	0.5	0.4
Soft drinks†	1.5	1.1	1.7	1.4	1.6	1.4
Fruit juice	0.4	0	0.4	0	0.3	0
Various sugary foods §	5.0	4.9	5.6	5.2	5.6	5.3
Average daily intake** of:						
Sugar confectionery (g)	5.9	0	10.0	4.3	12.2	5.7
Chocolate confectionery(g)	8.4	4.9	11.7	8.6	11.7	8.5
Soft drinks† (g)	229	145	268	191	278	226
Fruit juice (g)	39	0	37.8	0	35.5	0
Various sugary foods § (g)	353	296	407	342	424	380
Average daily intake†† (g) of:						
Total sugars	80.6	77.1	88.5	87.0	93.3	91.2
Non-milk extrinsic sugars	48.6	43.3	59.3	55.6	64.5	60.6
Intrinsic and milk sugars and starch	89.7	87.5	97.2	97.0	105	103
Carbohydrate	139	134	157	155	170	168
Base		*465*		*566*		*537*

* Median values of 0 show that over 50% of children did not consume the food.
† Includes fruit squashes with sugar, and carbonated drinks.
§ Includes intakes from the following food groups: biscuits; buns, cakes, pastries; fruit pies; milk, sponge and other puddings; ice cream; yogurt; fruit in syrup; sugar; preserves; sugar confectionery; chocolate confectionery; fruit juice; other soft drinks.
** Weight of sugary products consumed (in grams).
†† Nutrient variable measuring actual intake of sugars/nutrients within all foods, including intakes from dietary supplements.

Table 5.25 Upper and lower percentiles for the frequency of consumption of selected foods containing sugars and the average daily intake of these foods and selected nutrients, by age

Weighed intake data

Average daily frequency of consumption of sugary foods and average daily intake of these foods and selected nutrients	Age of child (in years)					
	1¹/₂- 2¹/₂		2¹/₂- 3¹/₂		3¹/₂- 4¹/₂	
Percentile	*10*	*90*	*10*	*90*	*10*	*90*
Average daily frequency of consumption of:						
Sugar confectionery	0	0.7	0	1.1	0	1.1
Chocolate confectionery	0	1.0	0	1.1	0	1.0
Soft drinks *	0	3.5	0	3.6	0	3.4
Fruit juice	0	1.4	0	1.2	0	1.1
Various sugary foods †	2.0	8.1	2.6	9.1	2.8	8.7
Average daily intake § of:						
Sugar confectionery (g)	0	21.1	0	29.5	0	35.7
Chocolate confectionery(g)	0	21.4	0	26.8	0	30.9
Soft drinks * (g)	0	565	0	615	0	604
Fruit juice (g)	0	139	0	138	0	112
Various sugary foods † (g)	71.2	697	118	754	132	740
Average daily intake (g) of:**						
Total sugars	48.2	116	54.9	125	57.9	134
Non-milk extrinsic sugars	20.4	82.7	28.9	95.5	32.2	104
Intrinsic and milk sugars and starch	61.8	120	66.3	126	75.8	139
Carbohydrate	97.7	182	111	200	126	219
Base		*465*		*566*		*537*

* Includes fruit squashes with sugar, and carbonated drinks.
† Includes intakes from the following food groups: biscuits; buns, cakes, pastries; fruit pies; milk, sponge and other puddings; ice cream; yogurt; fruit in syrup; sugar; preserves; sugar confectionery; chocolate confectionery; fruit juice; other soft drinks .
§ Weight of sugary products consumed (in grams).
** Nutrient variable measuring actual intake of sugars/nutrients within all foods, including intakes from dietary supplements.

An attempt was made to measure the frequency of consumption of sugary foods as frequent exposure to sugars as well as a high intake is known to be related to dental caries.[12] When interpreting the data relating to the frequency of consumption of different foods it is important to know the way in which the variables for frequency of consumption were calculated. Calculations were based on the number of entries of the relevant food codes in the four-day diary, weighted to give an average daily frequency. Limitations arise due to the fact that a mother who gave her child a drink containing sugars in the morning would probably have recorded it as one entry, but the child might have sipped at the drink over a period of several hours, rather than consume it immediately. Ideally information about such patterns of consumption would have been recorded, but this was beyond the scope of this study.

According to the data as calculated, on average, 1¹/₂ to 2¹/₂ year olds consumed sugars, in the form of the sugary foods listed, five times a day and those in the older two age cohorts consumed sugary foods 5.6 times a day (mean values from Table 5.24). The lowest consuming 10% of children had sugars from the food groups selected fewer than three times a day; the highest 10% had sugars from these sources more than eight times a day (Table 5.25).

The mean average daily intake of sugary foods ranged from 353g among 1¹/₂ to 2¹/₂ year olds, to 424g for children aged

3¹/₂ to 4¹/₂ years (Table 5.24). These figures represent the total weight of the foods from the sugary foods groups.

The average daily intake of total sugars shows the actual quantity of sugar obtained from all food sources. The mean intakes ranged from 80.6g among 1¹/₂ to 2¹/₂ year olds to 93.3g among 3¹/₂ to 4¹/₂ year olds. Total sugars can be classified as 'intrinsic and milk sugars' and 'non-milk extrinsic' (NME) sugars;[4] the latter are considered to be particularly damaging to the teeth.[5] Intakes of NME sugars ranged from 48.6g among 1¹/₂ to 2¹/₂ year olds to 64.5g among 3¹/₂ to 4¹/₂ year olds (Table 5.24). On average children in each age cohort were receiving 29% of their total energy intake from all sugars and 17% (1¹/₂ to 2¹/₂ years) to 20% (3¹/₂ to 4¹/₂ years) from NME sugars; for the population as a whole it is recommended that NME sugars should contribute no more than an average of 10% of total dietary energy[13] (tables not shown).

5.8 Household expenditure on sweets and chocolates

In the dental interview, parents were asked to estimate their weekly household expenditure on chocolates and sweets. This measure can be used as an indicator of the quantity of sweets that might be accessible to the child. Overall 3% of children lived in households where no money was spent on confectionery and 8% lived in households where expenditure on chocolates and sweets exceeded £5 a week. Half the children lived in households where some money, but less than £2 a week was spent on chocolates and sweets and the remaining 38% lived in households which spent an average of £2 to £5 on confectionery each week (Table 5.26). Significant variations in household expenditure on confectionery were found for manual and non-manual households (Table 5.27). For example, 5% of non-manual households reported spending more than £5 a week on chocolates and sweets on average, compared with 11% of manual households (p<0.01).

Table 5.26 Average weekly household expenditure on chocolates and sweets, by age

Average weekly household expenditure on chocolates and sweets	Age of child (in years)			
	$1^1/_2$ - $2^1/_2$	$2^1/_2$ - $3^1/_2$	$3^1/_2$ - $4^1/_2$	All ages
	%	%	%	%
Nothing	3	3	3	3
Less than £2 a week	53	49	50	50
£2 to £5 a week	36	40	38	38
More than £5 a week	8	8	9	8
Base	*497*	*598*	*559*	*1654*

Table 5.27 Average weekly household expenditure on chocolates and sweets, by social class of head of household and age of child

Social class of head of household and average weekly household expenditure on chocolates and sweets	Age of child (in years)			
	$1^1/_2$ - $2^1/_2$	$2^1/_2$ - $3^1/_2$	$3^1/_2$ - $4^1/_2$	All ages
	%	%	%	%
Non-manual				
Nothing	4	5	4	5
Less than £2 a week	60	56	59	58
£2 to £5 a week	27	35	34	32
More than £5 a week	8	3	3	5
Base	*226*	*268*	*246*	*740*
Manual				
Nothing	2	2	1	2
Less than £2 a week	47	42	43	44
£2 to £5 a week	43	45	43	43
More than £5 a week	7	11	13	11
Base	*250*	*308*	*296*	*854*

References and notes

1 The term dinky feeder used in this Report refers to the small comforter a child can be given, with a reservoir feeder for small quantities of liquid behind the teat.

2 The data relating to past users of bottles could be used for modelling, enabling the age at which bottle usage started and stopped and the drinks consumed from bottles during the day and at night to be related to data from the dental examination. Such modelling is beyond the scope of this Report, however the data tapes will be lodged at the ESRC archive at Essex University and future analysts may examine these issues.

3 Diet carbonated drinks were included with the group of drinks containing non-milk extrinsic sugars because their acidic content is thought to contribute to dental caries and erosion.

4 Sugars may be classified as intrinsic or extrinsic:
Extrinsic sugars are not located within the cellular structure of food, they are either free in food or added to it. Extrinsic sugars are further classified as
   - *milk sugars* (mainly lactose) naturally occurring in milk and milk products
   - *non-milk extrinsic sugars*
Intrinsic sugars are naturally integrated into the cellular structure of a food. The most important sources are whole fruits and vegetables containing mainly fructose, glucose and sucrose. Definitions taken from note 5.

5 Department of Health *Dietary Sugars and Human Disease.* HMSO (1989). Report on Health and Social Subjects:37.

6 A feeder beaker is a cup with a lid incorporating a spout, also known as a training beaker.

7 Rugg-Gunn A J. Diet and Dental Caries. In: Murray J J ed*The prevention of dental disease* 2nd edition. Oxford University Press, 1989.

8 A page of the diary is shown at Appendix B.

9 The nutrient database will be deposited with the survey data files at the ESRC archive at Essex University. Additional information about the contents of the database is included in the dietary survey report.[11]

10 The method of weighting is explained in more detail in Appendix J of the NDNS diet and nutrition report.[11]

11 Gregory J R Collins D L Davies P S W Hughes J M Clarke P C. National Diet and Nutrition Survey: children aged $1^1/_2$ to $4^1/_2$ years. Volume 1: *Report of the diet and nutrition survey.* HMSO (1995).

12 Shaw J H Diet and Dental Health *The American Journal of Clinical Nutrition 41*: May 1985 pp1117-1131.

13 Department of Health *Weaning and the Weaning Diet.* HMSO (1994). Report on Health and Social Subjects:45.

6 Variations in patterns of decay

Summary of chapter

This chapter considers relationships between a wide range of measures of dental care and dental decay, and between dietary practices *at the time of interview* and dental decay. Multi-variate analysis was carried out to identify the factors which had the strongest relationships with caries, independently of other measures. This analysis included characteristics of children and their families.

Dental care and dietary variables strongly associated with decay experience

Children who started having their teeth brushed, or who were brushing their own teeth before the age of one year were significantly less likely to have experience of dental decay than those who started toothbrushing later.

The frequency of toothbrushing was also associated with decay experience, with the group of children whose teeth were brushed more than once a day having less experience of decay than those where brushing was less frequent.

Children who always brushed their own teeth were more likely to have decay than those who sometimes or always had their teeth brushed by an adult.

Having a drink in bed every night, at the time of the survey, was associated with having tooth decay among children aged $1^1/_2$ to $2^1/_2$ and $2^1/_2$ to $3^1/_2$ years and if the drink consumed in bed contained non-milk extrinsic sugars, the likelihood of experiencing dental decay increased further.

The proportion of children with tooth decay among those who consumed sugar confectionery on most days of the week or more often was double the proportion among those who consumed sugar confectionery less frequently. Frequent consumption of carbonated drinks was also related to experience of dental decay.

A strong relationship was found between household expenditure on confectionery and dental decay among children aged $1^1/_2$ to $4^1/_2$ years.

Variables found to be independently related to decay experience

The *main* discriminator between children with and without experience of decay was, for $1^1/_2$ to $2^1/_2$ year olds, whether or not their parents were in receipt of Income Support or Family Credit; for $2^1/_2$ to $3^1/_2$ year olds, their mother's highest educational qualification, and for $3^1/_2$ to $4^1/_2$ year olds, the social class of the head of the household. After controlling for the effects of these variables, further independent relationships were as follows:

- for $1^1/_2$ to $2^1/_2$ year olds, who brushed their teeth
- for $2^1/_2$ to $3^1/_2$ year olds, usually having a drink containing non-milk extrinsic sugars in bed
- for $3^1/_2$ to $4^1/_2$ year olds, in descending order of importance, the region of Britain in which they lived, household expenditure on confectionery and whether their parents were receiving Income Support or Family Credit.

Therefore, despite strong relationships between measures of dental hygiene (especially toothbrushing) and dental decay, and despite higher levels of decay among children who for example were reported to be high consumers of sugars, background factors were more powerful discriminators between children with and without experience of dental caries.

6.1 Introduction

The decay experience of children from different backgrounds was compared in Chapter 3. In this chapter, decay experience is shown in relation to other factors, mainly behavioural, which were thought to affect the likelihood of children experiencing dental decay. These factors include children's dental care practices and dietary habits which were discussed in Chapters 4 and 5.

The majority of tables in this chapter present the proportions of children with active decay, filled teeth, missing teeth and any decay experience in relation to variables associated with dental care and dietary practice. Where the behaviour measured by a variable is strongly associated with age, for example visiting the dentist, the tables show data for children in the three age cohorts only, excluding 'all children'.

The mean numbers of teeth with decay experience in relation to the dental care and dietary behaviour variables are shown in Appendix D.

Inter-relationships were thought to exist between some of the measures of dental care and dietary practice shown in this chapter. Multi-variate analysis was therefore undertaken to identify factors which had independent relationships with dental decay; the results are presented in section 6.4.

6.2 Measures associated with dental care

6.2.1 Toothbrushing

The younger children were when they started toothbrushing, the lower the proportion having tooth decay. Overall, 12% of children who started toothbrushing before the age of one year were found to have some experience of decay, compared with 19% of those who started between the ages of one and two years and 34% of those who did not start toothbrushing until after the age of 2 years (p<0.01). *(Table 6.1)*

The frequency with which children's teeth were reported to be brushed was also associated with dental decay experience for children in each age cohort. Among the group aged $3\frac{1}{2}$ to $4\frac{1}{2}$ years, 24% of children whose teeth were brushed more than once a day had experience of dental decay compared with 38% of those whose teeth were brushed once a day (p<0.05) and almost half (48%) of those whose teeth were brushed less often (p<0.05). *(Table 6.2)*

Compared with children whose teeth were currently always or sometimes brushed by an adult, children who brushed their own teeth had higher prevalence of dental decay (Table 6.3). The differences were most noticeable in the youngest age cohort where 7% of children who always brushed their own teeth had experience of decay, compared with only 1% of those where toothbrushing was shared between the child and an adult and 4% among children whose teeth were brushed by an adult only (differences not significant, p>0.05).

As was reported in Chapter 4, some of the children who currently brushed their own teeth, had never had their teeth brushed by an adult; among $3\frac{1}{2}$ to $4\frac{1}{2}$ year olds who had only ever brushed their own teeth, almost half (48%) had experience of caries and 11% had had an extraction (n=54)(table not shown). Despite the small base, the difference in caries experience between this group and the group of children where toothbrushing was shared between an adult and child was statistically significant (p<0.05; 28% of $3\frac{1}{2}$ to $4\frac{1}{2}$ year olds whose teeth were sometimes brushed by an adult and sometimes by a child had dental decay experience).

6.2.2 Visits to the dentist

Among children aged 5 to 15 years there is a strong relationship between dental attendance patterns and dental decay,[1] with children who regularly visit the dentist having less dental decay than those who go occasionally, or only when they have trouble with their teeth. For children aged $1\frac{1}{2}$ to

Table 6.1 Proportion of children with any active decay, filled teeth, teeth missing due to decay and any decay experience, by age and age when started toothbrushing

Age when started toothbrushing and type of decay	Age of child (in years)			
	$1\frac{1}{2}$ - $2\frac{1}{2}$	$2\frac{1}{2}$ - $3\frac{1}{2}$	$3\frac{1}{2}$ - $4\frac{1}{2}$	All ages
	Percentage of children with each type of decay			
Less than one year				
Active decay	3	9	20	11
Filled teeth	0	0	2	1
Teeth missing due to decay	0	1	2	1
Any decay experience	3	10	22	12
Base	*247*	*265*	*250*	*762*
One year to two years				
Active decay	4	15	34	18
Filled teeth	0	1	7	3
Teeth missing due to decay	1	0	4	1
Any decay experience	4	15	37	19
Base	*180*	*218*	*200*	*598*
Over two years				
Active decay	[0]	29	37	32
Filled teeth	[0]	2	5	4
Teeth missing due to decay	[0]	2	9	6
Any decay experience	[0]	29	39	34
Base	*5*	*49*	*79*	*133*

Table 6.2 Proportion of children with any active decay, filled teeth, teeth missing due to decay and any decay experience, by age and frequency of toothbrushing

Frequency of toothbrushing and type of decay	Age of child (in years)			
	$1\frac{1}{2}$ - $2\frac{1}{2}$	$2\frac{1}{2}$ - $3\frac{1}{2}$	$3\frac{1}{2}$ - $4\frac{1}{2}$	All ages
	Percentage of children with each type of decay			
Less than once a day				
Active decay	9	22	48	25
Filled teeth	0	2	6	2
Teeth missing due to decay	0	3	6	3
Any decay experience	9	23	48	26
Base	*58*	*64*	*52*	*174*
Once a day				
Active decay	2	14	34	16
Filled teeth	0	0	6	2
Teeth missing due to decay	0	0	4	1
Any decay experience	2	14	38	18
Base	*171*	*174*	*161*	*506*
More than once a day				
Active decay	4	11	22	13
Filled teeth	0	1	3	2
Teeth missing due to decay	0	0	3	1
Any decay experience	4	12	24	14
Base	*222*	*301*	*323*	*846*

Table 6.3 Proportion of children with any active decay, filled teeth, teeth missing due to decay and any decay experience, by age and who brushes child's teeth

Who brushes child's teeth and type of decay	Age of child (in years)		
	$1^1/_2$ - $2^1/_2$	$2^1/_2$ - $3^1/_2$	$3^1/_2$ - $4^1/_2$
	Percentage of children with each type of decay		
Child brushes own teeth			
Active decay	7	15	32
Filled teeth	0	1	3
Teeth missing due to decay	0	1	4
Any decay experience	7	15	34
Base	*122*	*159*	*206*
Adult brushes child's teeth			
Active decay	4	11	29
Filled teeth	0	0	2
Teeth missing due to decay	0	1	4
Any decay experience	4	11	30
Base	*140*	*124*	*100*
Varies - adult or child			
Active decay	1	13	24
Filled teeth	0	1	6
Teeth missing due to decay	1	0	3
Any decay experience	1	14	28
Base	*171*	*252*	*227*

Table 6.4 Proportion of children with any active decay, filled teeth, teeth missing due to decay and any decay experience, by age and child's experience of visiting the dentist

Visits to the dentist and type of decay	Age of child (in years)		
	$1^1/_2$ - $2^1/_2$	$2^1/_2$ - $3^1/_2$	$3^1/_2$ - $4^1/_2$
	Percentage of children with each type of decay		
Seen and examined			
Active decay	5	14	26
Filled teeth	0	1	6
Teeth missing due to decay	1	1	5
Any decay experience	6	15	30
Base	*110*	*286*	*413*
Seen but not examined			
Active decay	2	7	25
Filled teeth	0	0	0
Teeth missing due to decay	0	0	0
Any decay experience	2	7	25
Base	*43*	*44*	*20*
Never seen a dentist			
Active decay	4	14	34
Filled teeth	0	0	0
Teeth missing due to decay	0	0	0
Any decay experience	4	14	34
Base	*297*	*211*	*103*

$4^1/_2$ years the information on dental attendance relates to whether children had ever been examined by a dentist, had seen a dentist without being examined, or had never seen a dentist (Table 6.4). Differences in active decay and total decay experience between children who had been seen and examined by a dentist and those who had never seen a dentist, were not statistically significant (p>0.05), although among $3^1/_2$ to $4^1/_2$ year olds, active decay appeared to affect a smaller proportion of those who had been seen and examined (26%), than of those who had never seen a dentist (34%). Among children who had been seen and examined by a dentist, some dental decay had been treated; for example, 6% of children aged $3^1/_2$ to $4^1/_2$ years who had been examined by a dentist had filled teeth and 5% had teeth missing due to decay.

6.2.3 Advice received by parents about caring for their child's teeth

Table 6.5 shows the proportion of children with decay experience in relation to advice received by their parents about their child's diet, toothbrushing, and the use of fluoride drops or tablets, referred to as fluoride supplements.[2] There was little difference in decay prevalence between children whose parents said they had and had not received the sorts of advice covered in the interview.

6.2.4 Use of fluoride supplements[2]

Parents may be advised to give their children fluoride drops

Table 6.5 Proportion of children with experience of decay according to whether advice on dental care received by parents, by age of child

Whether different types of advice received	Age of child (in years)							
	$1^1/_2$ - $2^1/_2$		$2^1/_2$ - $3^1/_2$		$3^1/_2$ - $4^1/_2$		All ages	
	%*	*Base*	%*	*Base*	%*	*Base*	%*	*Base*
Received advice on:								
Food and drink	3	*184*	17	*213*	32	*241*	19	*638*
Toothbrushing	2	*106*	13	*162*	30	*200*	17	*468*
Giving fluoride	3	*98*	20	*121*	33	*129*	20	*348*
Not giving fluoride	7	*44*	9	*54*	18	*49*	12	*147*
No advice on:								
Food and drink	5	*267*	12	*328*	29	*295*	15	*890*
Toothbrushing	5	*345*	14	*379*	31	*336*	16	*1060*
Giving fluoride	4	*353*	12	*418*	29	*407*	16	*1178*
Not giving fluoride	4	*407*	14	*486*	31	*486*	17	*1379*
Received some advice	2	*252*	15	*323*	30	*352*	17	*927*
Received advice on none of above	6	*199*	12	*217*	30	*184*	16	*600*

* This table shows the percentage of children with any decay experience; each percentage is calculated on the base shown in the right hand column. The column percentages do not total 100%

or tablets for different reasons and they may be introduced at different ages. While some children use fluoride supplements before their deciduous teeth have erupted, in other cases they are not introduced until some dental caries has been found in the deciduous dentition. As was shown in Chapter 4 (sections 4.3.1 and 4.6.3), parents of children in Scotland were far more likely than those elsewhere in Britain to have been advised to give, and to have given their children fluoride supplements.

The varying patterns of use of fluoride supplements should be borne in mind when interpreting the differences in dental health that were found between children who had used fluoride supplements and those who had never used them (Table 6.6). Overall the users of supplements had more dental decay, with 22% of supplement users having some decay experience compared with 15% of non-supplement users (p<0.05). When the age at which children started using fluoride supplements was considered in relation to decay experience (Table 6.7), it can be seen that among children who were given fluoride supplements before the age of one, decay levels were almost identical to those for all children in the survey. However, among children who started using fluoride supplements aged one year or over, decay levels were considerably higher than for the population in general.

6.2.5 Mothers dental attendance pattern

Chapter 4 showed a relationship between the dental attendance patterns of children's mothers, and their child going to the dentist. This measure may also reflect other general attitudes towards dental care. Table 6.8 shows a greater prevalence of decay experience among children whose mothers reported only going to the dentist when having trouble with their teeth than among the children of regular attenders. Among $3^1/_2$ to $4^1/_2$ year olds for example, decay experience affected 45% of children whose mothers visited the dentist only when they had dental trouble, compared with only 25% of those whose mothers regularly visited the dentist (p<0.01).

Table 6.6 Proportion of children with any active decay, filled teeth, teeth missing due to decay and any decay experience, by age and use of fluoride supplements

Use of fluoride supplements and type of decay	Age of child (in years)			
	$1^1/_2$ - $2^1/_2$	$2^1/_2$ - $3^1/_2$	$3^1/_2$ - $4^1/_2$	All ages
	Percentage of children with each type of decay			
Child has used fluoride supplements				
Active decay	4	21	30	20
Filled teeth	0	3	8	4
Teeth missing due to decay	0	1	7	3
Any decay experience	4	22	33	22
Base	*72*	*98*	*111*	*281*
Child has never used fluoride supplements				
Active decay	4	12	27	15
Filled teeth	0	0	3	1
Teeth missing due to decay	0	0	3	1
Any decay experience	4	12	29	15
Base	*379*	*442*	*425*	*1246*

Table 6.7 Proportion of children with any active decay, filled teeth, teeth missing due to decay and any decay experience, by age and age started using fluoride supplements

Age started using fluoride and type of decay	Age of child (in years)			
	$1^1/_2$ - $2^1/_2$	$2^1/_2$ - $3^1/_2$	$3^1/_2$ - $4^1/_2$	All ages
	Percentage of children with each type of decay			
Started using fluoride supplements before age of 1 year				
Active decay	4	15	27	15
Filled teeth	0	5	5	3
Teeth missing due to decay	0	2	7	3
Any decay experience	4	17	32	18
Base	*54*	*65*	*56*	*175*
Started using fluoride supplements aged 1 year and over				
Active decay	[1]	35	34	30
Filled teeth	[0]	0	11	6
Teeth missing due to decay	[0]	0	3	4
Any decay experience	[1]	35	36	31
Base	*17*	*31*	*53*	*101*
All children				
Active decay	4	13	28	16
Filled teeth	0	1	4	2
Teeth missing due to decay	0	1	4	2
Any decay experience	4	14	30	17
Base	*451*	*544*	*537*	*1532*

Table 6.8 Proportion of children with any active decay, filled teeth, teeth missing due to decay and any decay experience, by age and mother's dental attendance pattern

Mother's dental attendance pattern and child's tooth condition	Age of child (in years)			
	$1^1/_2$ - $2^1/_2$	$2^1/_2$ - $3^1/_2$	$3^1/_2$ - $4^1/_2$	All ages
	Percentage of children with each type of decay			
Regular				
Active decay	2	12	23	13
Filled teeth	0	1	4	2
Teeth missing due to decay	0	1	4	2
Any decay experience	3	12	25	15
Base	*259*	*332*	*338*	*919*
Occasional				
Active decay	8	14	26	16
Filled teeth	0	0	3	1
Teeth missing due to decay	0	0	3	1
Any decay experience	8	14	27	16
Base	*73*	*66*	*66*	*205*
Trouble				
Active decay	5	17	41	21
Filled teeth	0	1	5	2
Teeth missing due to decay	0	1	3	1
Any decay experience	5	17	45	22
Base	*109*	*142*	*121*	*372*

6.3 Measures associated with eating and drinking and dental condition

6.3.1 The use of bottles, dinky feeders and dummies

Overall, children who had used a bottle, dinky feeder or dummy had more chance of having dental decay than other children; 32% of those who had used one of the above had experience of caries compared with 13% of those who had not (p<0.01). Among $3^{1}/_{2}$ to $4^{1}/_{2}$ year olds, comparing decay among users and non-users, the use of bottles and dinky feeders was more strongly related to decay than was the use of dummies; for example, 32% of bottle users had caries experience compared with 17% of those who had never used a bottle (p<0.05).   (*Table 6.9*)

6.3.2 Night-time drinking and eating practices at the time of interview

Table 6.10 shows a range of measures relating dental decay experience to having drinks in bed or during the night. Among children aged $1^{1}/_{2}$ to $2^{1}/_{2}$ years and $2^{1}/_{2}$ to $3^{1}/_{2}$ years a higher proportion of those who had drinks every night had decay experience than of those who had drinks in bed only sometimes, or never. For example, 21% of $2^{1}/_{2}$ to $3^{1}/_{2}$ year olds who had a drink in bed every night had experience of decay compared with 8% of those who sometimes had a drink in bed (p<0.05) and 12% of those who never had a drink in bed (p>0.05). Among children aged $3^{1}/_{2}$ to $4^{1}/_{2}$ years the data suggest that a smaller proportion of children who had a drink in bed every night had dental decay than was found among those who never had a drink in bed, however this apparent difference was not statistically significant (p<0.05). Due to the fact that children's current practice may not reflect their behaviour at a younger age, relating measures such as having a drink in bed at the time of interview to dental decay is more reliable among younger than older children.

A significantly higher proportion of children who consumed drinks containing non-milk extrinsic (NME) sugars[3] in bed, had tooth decay (26%) than did children who drank milk (12%) or water (11%) in bed (p<0.01). Among children who consumed drinks in bed every night, 29% of those who had a drink containing, NME sugars had experience of decay compared with 11% of those who had milk (p<0.01). The classification of drinks is shown as note 4 to this chapter.
                                                        (*Table 6.10*)

Differences were found in the proportion of children with experience of decay depending on the type of drinking vessel usually used at night. For each age cohort, decay experience appeared to affect a higher proportion of bottle users than of those using other vessels, however the numbers of children in each group were generally small and apparent differences were not significant (p>0.05) (Table 6.10). Among $3^{1}/_{2}$ to $4^{1}/_{2}$ year olds for example, 42% of those still using bottles in bed had experience of decay compared with only 28% of those using a mug, cup or glass. The drinks consumed from different vessels at night are shown in Chapter 5 (Table 5.15).

Chapter 5 showed that very few children in the survey were said ever to eat anything in bed at night. Overall, 26% of the 69 children who sometimes ate in bed had experience of caries compared with 16% among those who did not (difference not significant, p>0.05, table not shown).

6.3.3 Household spending on confectionery

Table 6.11 shows a strong relationship between average weekly household expenditure on chocolates and sweets and dental decay. Among children aged $3^{1}/_{2}$ to $4^{1}/_{2}$ years, 20% of those whose parents spent less than £2 a week on confectionery had decay experience compared with 38% of those whose parents spent between £2 and £5 a week and 60% of those whose parents spent more than £5 each week (p<0.01).

6.3.4 Dietary measures and dental condition

This section presents some data relating dental decay to dietary habits. When interpreting the results it is important to bear in mind the nature of the survey data. The dietary information showed the diet at a fixed point in time, but dental decay develops over time and it is unlikely that children's diets recorded at the time of the survey, were the same as their diets over their lifetimes. Indeed, the presence of tooth decay could be a factor causing dietary change. It is also important to remember that dietary habits are only one

Table 6.9 Proportion of children with any decay experience by age and whether used a bottle, dinky feeder, or dummy

Use of bottles, dinky-feeders and dummies	Age of child (in years)							
	$1^{1}/_{2}$ - $2^{1}/_{2}$		$2^{1}/_{2}$ - $3^{1}/_{2}$		$3^{1}/_{2}$ - $4^{1}/_{2}$		All ages	
	%*	Base	%*	Base	%*	Base	%*	Base
All children	4	451	14	514	30	537	17	1532
Use of bottle								
Yes	4	401	14	474	32	466	17	1341
No	6	50	12	67	17	70	12	187
Use of dinky-feeder								
Yes	4	79	11	101	39	99	19	279
No	4	372	15	440	28	437	16	1249
Use of dummy								
Yes	4	252	16	282	32	287	18	821
No	4	199	12	259	28	249	15	707
Use of any comforter above								
Yes	4	415	14	488	32	481	32	1384
No	3	36	15	37	16	38	13	144

* This table shows the percentage of children with any decay experience; each percentage is calculated on the base shown in the right hand column. The column percentages do not total 100%.

Table 6.10 Proportion of children with any decay experience by age and night-time drinking practices at the time of interview

Type of night-time drinking practice	Age of child (in years)							
	1½ - 2½		2½ - 3½		3½ - 4½		All ages	
	%*	Base	%*	Base	%*	Base	%*	Base
All children	4	451	14	514	30	537	17	1532
Frequency of drinking in bed								
Every night	6	183	21	171	26	117	16	471
Some nights, but not every night	0	52	8	89	31	118	17	259
Never	3	216	12	281	32	301	17	798
When drink in bed, type of drink consumed								
Drink containing NME sugars	9	55	28	60	38	64	26	179
Milk	4	130	14	87	28	47	12	237
Water	0	34	8	53	19	74	11	161
If drink in bed every night, usual drink								
Drink containing NME sugars	12	41	40	40	35	37	29	118
Milk	4	90	15	68	19	31	11	189
Vessel usually used when drink at night								
Bottle	7	151	21	92	42	33	†	†
Feeder beaker	2	57	18	82	18	51	†	†
Mug, cup or glass	[0]	16	10	49	28	148	†	†

* This table shows the percentage of children with any decay experience; each percentage is calculated on the base shown in the right hand column.
The column percentages do not total 100%.

† This analysis was only carried out for individual age groups.

Table 6.11 Proportion of children with any active decay, filled teeth, teeth missing due to decay and any decay experience, by age and average weekly household expenditure on chocolates and sweets

Average weekly household expenditure on chocolates and sweets and type of decay	Age of child (in years)			
	1½ - 2½	2½ - 3½	3½ - 4½	All ages
	Percentage of children with each type of decay			
Less than £2				
Active decay	3	11	18	11
Filled teeth	0	1	3	1
Teeth missing due to decay	0	1	4	1
Any decay experience	3	13	20	12
Base	250	280	282	812
£2 to £5				
Active decay	4	16	36	19
Filled teeth	0	0	4	2
Teeth missing due to decay	1	0	3	2
Any decay experience	5	16	38	20
Base	163	218	203	584
Over £5				
Active decay	8	12	54	27
Filled teeth	0	0	14	5
Teeth missing due to decay	0	0	6	2
Any decay experience	8	12	60	30
Base	37	42	50	129

set of factors contributing to dental decay and causal relationships between diet and caries may therefore be confused by differences in dental practices which are unrelated to diet. As behaviour changes over time, caution is particularly necessary when examining relationships between current dietary habits and dental decay among older children.

(i) Consumption of foods containing sugars, as reported in the dietary interview (food frequency questions) and decay experience

Tables 6.12 and 6.13 show decay experience for children in the three age cohorts in relation to the frequency of consumption, at the time of interview, of a range of foods and drinks (the frequency of consumption of the foods considered are shown in Chapter 5; Tables 5.20 to 5.22). In order to provide sufficient cases for comparison, it has been necessary to group frequencies of consumption. For children of all ages the frequency of consumption of sugar confectionery (Table 6.12) was related to dental decay; for example, 40% of 3½ to 4½ year olds who were reported to have sugar confectionery most days or more often had experience of caries compared with 22% of those who consumed sugar confectionery less frequently, or never ($p < 0.01$). Children who consumed carbonated drinks (including low-calorie carbonated drinks) most days or more often were also considerably more likely to have tooth decay than those who consumed carbonated drinks less frequently (Table 6.13). For example, of 2½ to 3½ year olds who had carbonated drinks most frequently, 22% had decay experience, double the proportion of less frequent consumers (11%) who were affected ($p < 0.05$).

For the other foods and drinks in Tables 6.12 and 6.13 strong relationships between frequency of consumption and dental decay were not found, or trends were not consistent across all age groups. Among older children it is particularly likely that dietary behaviour at the time of interview might be different from that earlier when any caries was developing.

(ii) Consumption of selected foods and nutrients (weighed intake data) and decay experience

Chapter 5 presented the mean and median frequency of consumption of selected foods containing sugars, and the average daily intake of these foods and selected nutrients for children in each age group. In this chapter, the same information is shown separately for children with and without caries experience[5]. This is only possible for children aged $2^1/_2$ to $3^1/_2$ years and $3^1/_2$ to $4^1/_2$ years, as too few children in the youngest age group had any decay experience (Tables 6.14 and 6.15). The tables show some apparent differences, but few of these reach statistical significance. The average daily frequency of consumption of the foods containing sugars listed, was very similar for the groups of children with and without caries. However, it appears that children with decay experience had higher average intakes of sugar confectionery and soft drinks (fruit squashes with sugar, and carbonated drinks, including low-calorie carbonated drinks) than those without caries experience. For example, among $2^1/_2$ to $3^1/_2$ year olds, the mean average daily intake of sugar confectionery was 14.7g for children with caries experience compared with 9.2g for those without caries experience. For fruit juice, the opposite trend was found, with the mean average daily intake for $3^1/_2$ to $4^1/_2$ year olds without caries experience (43.4g), significantly higher than that for children

with experience of caries, (15.0g, p<0.01). Consumption of fruit juice was far more common among children from non-manual backgrounds than among those from households with a manual head,[6] and as has already been shown (Section 3.2.2), a significantly lower proportion of children from non-manual backgrounds had experience of dental decay than from manual backgrounds.

To investigate further possible relationships between dietary behaviour and dental health, the children with the most extreme consumption patterns were compared. Table 6.16 shows the proportions of children with caries among the 10% consuming certain foods containing sugars least and most frequently (columns headed 10 and 90 respectively) and among the 10% with the lowest and highest intakes of these foods and certain nutrients.[7] For this analysis commentary is confined to the data for children aged $1^1/_2$ to $2^1/_2$ years as their dietary habits at the time of interview were more likely to reflect practices at the time when any caries developed than were the current diets of older children. Among these youngest children, for almost all of the foods and nutrients listed, the groups with the highest consumption appear to have higher decay prevalence than the groups with the lowest consumption, however these apparent differences are not statistically significant (p>0.05). It is interesting to note that none of the 10% of $1^1/_2$ to $2^1/_2$ year olds with the lowest average daily intake of NME sugars had experience of dental caries, compared with 8% of those with the highest average daily intakes of NME sugars. NME sugars are thought to be particularly cariogenic.[8]

Table 6.12 Proportion of children with experience of decay by age and the frequency with which they were reported to consume various foods containing sugars

Food frequency data

Frequency of consuming sugar confectionery, chocolate confectionery, biscuits, cakes and ice creams or ice lollies	Age of child (in years)					
	$1^1/_2$ - $2^1/_2$		$2^1/_2$ - $3^1/_2$		$3^1/_2$ - $4^1/_2$	
	%*	Base	%*	Base	%*	Base
Proportion of all children with experience of decay	4	451	17	514	30	537
Sugar confectionery						
Most days or more often	6	147	18	254	40	255
Less frequently than most days†	3	304	10	289	22	281
Chocolate confectionery						
Once a day or more often	5	64	13	100	30	93
Most days	2	87	15	136	37	110
At least once a week	5	228	13	247	28	260
Less frequently than at least once a week†	1	70	15	60	29	73
Biscuits						
More than once a day	11	93	14	114	30	115
Once a day	5	103	15	118	31	108
Most days	1	166	14	204	31	209
Less frequently than most days†	1	87	12	108	27	105
Cakes						
Most days or more often	4	53	14	85	27	81
At least once a week	5	243	13	306	30	300
At least once a month	4	91	17	100	39	97
Less than once a month†	2	64	12	52	21	58
Ice cream or ice lollies						
Most days or more often	6	147	18	254	40	255
At least once a week	4	154	10	181	22	219
At least once a month	3	37	15	48	[4]	29
Less than once a month†	2	113	8	60	24	33

* This table shows the percentage of children with any decay experience;each percentage is calculated on the base shown in the right hand column.
  The column percentages do not total 100%. † Including non-consumers.

Table 6.13 Proportion of children with experience of decay by age and the frequency with which they were reported to consume various drinks containing sugars

Food frequency data

Frequency of consuming carbonated drinks, blackcurrant drinks and fruit juice	Age of child (in years)					
	$1^1/_2$ - $2^1/_2$		$2^1/_2$- $3^1/_2$		$3^1/_2$ - $4^1/_2$	
	%*	Base	%*	Base	%*	Base
Proportion of all children with experience of decay	4	451	17	514	30	537
Carbonated drinks †						
Most days or more often	4	75	22	143	44	157
Less often than most days**	4	376	11	400	25	379
Blackcurrant drinks§						
More than once a day	5	64	14	80	17	84
Once a day or most days	3	63	23	83	32	87
At least once a week	2	45	13	60	29	66
Sometimes but less frequently than at least once a week	5	78	7	98	28	117
Never	4	200	14	222	37	183
Fruit juice						
Once a day or more often	7	92	15	113	19	95
Most days	3	64	14	78	28	71
At least once a week	0	81	12	109	27	122
At least once a month	6	54	5	59	39	70
Less than once a month	0	32	9	43	37	43
Never	6	128	20	142	36	134

* This table shows the percentage of children with any decay experience; each percentage is calculated on the base shown in the right hand column. The column percentages do not total 100%.
† Including low-calorie carbonated drinks.
§ Including low-calorie blackcurrant drinks.
** Including those who never consume carbonated drinks.

Table 6.14 Average daily frequency of consumption of selected foods containing sugars, and average daily intake of these foods and selected nutrients, for children with and without experience of caries; children aged $2^1/_2$ to $3^1/_2$ years

Weighed intake data

Average daily frequency of consumption of sugary foods and average daily intake of these foods and selected nutrients	Children aged $2^1/_2$ to $3^1/_2$ years			
	Caries experience		No caries experience	
	Mean	Median*	Mean	Median*
Average daily frequency of consumption of:				
Sugar confectionery	0.5	0.4	0.4	0.1
Chocolate confectionery	0.5	0.4	0.5	0.4
Soft drinks†	1.8	1.2	1.7	1.4
Fruit juice	0.4	0	0.3	0
Various sugary foods§	5.5	4.4	5.6	5.4
Average daily intake of:**				
Sugar confectionery (g)	14.7	9.1	9.2	3.6
Chocolate confectionery (g)	11.3	8.2	11.8	8.7
Soft drinks†(g)	293	222	266	191
Fruit juice (g)	34.7	0	35.8	0
Various sugary foods§ (g)	427	366	403	334
Average daily intake †† (g) of:				
Total sugars	88.2	84.2	88.7	87.1
Non-milk extrinsic sugars	60.5	56.6	58.9	55.2
Intrinsic and milk sugars and starch	94.8	90.8	98.1	97.8
Carbohydrate	156	158	157	155
Base		70		443

* Median values of 0 show that over 50% of children did not consume the food.
† Includes fruit squashes with sugar, and carbonated drinks (including low-calorie carbonated drinks).
§ Includes intakes from the following food groups: biscuits; buns, cakes, pastries; fruit pies; milk, sponge and other puddings; ice cream; yogurt; fruit in syrup; sugar; preserves; sugar confectionery; chocolate confectionery; fruit juice; other soft drinks.
** Weight of sugary products consumed (in grams).
†† Nutrient variable measuring actual intake of sugars/nutrients within all foods, including intakes from dietary supplements.

Table 6.15 Average daily frequency of consumption of selected foods containing sugars and average daily intake of these foods and selected nutrients, for children with and without experience of caries; children aged 3½ to 4½ years

Weighed intake data

Average daily frequency of consumption of sugary foods and average daily intake of these foods and selected nutrients	Child's experience of caries at age 3½ to 4½ years			
	Caries experience		No caries experience	
	Mean	Median*	Mean	Median*
Average daily frequency of consumption of:				
Sugar confectionery	0.5	0.4	0.4	0.3
Chocolate confectionery	0.5	0.4	0.4	0.4
Soft drinks†	1.6	1.5	1.6	1.3
Fruit juice	0.1	0	0.4	0
Various sugary foods§	5.5	5.1	5.6	5.3
Average daily intakeof:**				
Sugar confectionery (g)	14.4	7.6	11.7	5.4
Chocolate confectionery (g)	13.0	9.3	11.3	7.9
Soft drinks†(g)	283	245	276	214
Fruit juice (g)	15.0	0	43.4	0
Various sugary foods§(g)	410	377	429	379
Average daily intake†† (g) of:				
Total sugars	93.0	91.3	93.5	91.0
Non-milk extrinsic sugars	65.3	64.7	64.3	59.2
Intrinsic and milk sugars and starch	105	100	105	105
Carbohydrate	171	162	169	169
Base		*154*		*361*

* Median values of 0 show that over 50% of children did not consume the food.
† Includes fruit squashes with sugar, and carbonated drinks (including low-calorie carbonated drinks).
§ Includes intakes from the following food groups: biscuits; buns, cakes, pastries; fruit pies; milk, sponge and other puddings; ice cream; yogurt; fruit in syrup; sugar; preserves; sugar confectionery; chocolate confectionery; fruit juice; other soft drinks.
** Weight of sugary products consumed (in grams).
†† Nutrient variable measuring actual intake of sugars/nutrients within all foods, including intakes from dietary supplements.

Table 6.16 Proportion of children with any decay experience for children whose average daily frequency of consumption and intakes of selected foods and nutrients, were below the 10th percentile value and above the 90th percentile value, by age

Weighed intake data

Frequency of consumption and average intakes of selected sugary foods and nutrients	Age of child (in years) and percentile											
	1½ - 2½				2½ - 3½				3½ - 4½			
	10		90		10		90		10		90	
	%	Base	%	Base	%	Base	%	Base	%	Base	%	Base
Average daily frequency of consumption of:												
Sugar confectionery	3	233	7	41	13	183	25	32	25	174	34	44
Chocolate confectionery	2	123	3	40	19	116	17	42	28	133	34	50
Soft drinks*	2	85	5	42	16	67	14	51	30	54	26	50
Fruit juice	4	276	3	37	15	338	8	48	36	325	9	46
Various sugary foods†	0	45	7	42	22	59	23	48	26	51	28	50
Average daily intake in grams§ of:												
Sugar confectionery	3	233	7	41	13	183	23	48	25	174	31	52
Chocolate confectionery	2	123	5	43	19	116	16	51	28	133	33	52
Soft drinks*	2	85	5	41	16	67	16	51	30	54	27	52
Fruit juice	4	276	3	38	15	338	13	48	36	325	8	51
Various sugary foods†	0	41	3	38	20	56	17	52	36	50	23	52
Average daily intake in grams of:**												
Total sugars	2	44	3	37	19	52	23	53	37	52	29	52
Non-milk extrinsic sugars	0	42	8	38	25	52	20	50	31	52	27	52
Intrinsic and milk sugars and starch	9	45	5	40	22	49	20	51	33	50	44	52
Carbohydrate	2	43	3	39	20	49	17	52	32	52	37	51

* Includes fruit squashes with sugar, and carbonated drinks (including low-calorie carbonated drinks).
† Includes intakes from the following food groups: biscuits; buns, cakes, pastries; fruit pies; milk, sponge and other puddings; ice cream; yogurt; fruit in syrup; sugar; preserves; sugar confectionery; chocolate confectionery; fruit juice; other soft drinks.
§ Weight of sugary products consumed.
** Nutrient variable measuring actual intake of sugars/nutrients within all foods, including intakes from dietary supplements

6.4 Independent relationships between behavioural variables and dental decay

Various behavioural factors have been shown to be associated with dental decay, but some of these factors are themselves inter-related. This section considers the combined effect of those behavioural variables found to have the strongest relationships with decay experience from Tables 6.1 to 6.16. A logistic regression model was run for two sets of behavioural variables separately; those relating to the consumption of foods containing sugars and to feeding practices, and those relating to dental care such as toothbrushing and visiting the dentist. Table 6.17 presents the findings of these analyses. The table lists the variables which were specified in the analysis, and identifies those which the model showed as being independently related to decay experience for each age group, in descending order of importance.[9] The background variables identified in Chapter 3 are also included in Table 6.17.

6.4.1 Dental care and dental decay

For the youngest children the major dental care variable associated with decay experience was who brushed the child's teeth. Among $2^1/_2$ to $3^1/_2$ year olds the age at which toothbrushing started was the main discriminator between children having and not having experience of caries. By the age of $3^1/_2$ to $4^1/_2$ years the frequency of toothbrushing was the most significant variable associated with dental decay, although the age at which toothbrushing started remained important, independent of the frequency of brushing. Mothers' dental attendance patterns were also independently re-

lated to children's experience of dental decay among $3^1/_2$ to $4^1/_2$ year olds.

6.4.2 Dietary behaviour and dental decay

Among $1^1/_2$ to $2^1/_2$ year olds and $2^1/_2$ to $3^1/_2$ year olds the main dietary measure differentiating between children with and without tooth decay was taking a drink containing NME sugars[3] to bed, as opposed to not drinking in bed or having other types of drink in bed. For children aged $2^1/_2$ to $3^1/_2$ years the frequency of consumption of carbonated drinks and average household spending on confectionery were also important. For children aged $3^1/_2$ to $4^1/_2$ years, household spending on confectionery, the frequency of having both carbonated drinks and sugar confectionery, and the use of a dinky feeder were all independently related to decay experience.

6.5 Independent relationships between background characteristics of children and their households, dental behaviour and dental decay

Multi-variate analysis was also carried out combining the behavioural variables and background variables which had been identified within their own groups as being independently related to decay experience to identify those which had the greatest effect overall and which independent relationships remained. *(Table 6.18)*

For each age group the most significant variable differentiating between children with and without experience of caries was a background characteristic. For children aged $1^1/_2$ to $2^1/_2$ years, whether the parents were in receipt of Income

Table 6.17 Background, dental care and dietary behaviour variables found to be independently related to decay, experience, by age

Variables put into model*	Age of child (in years)		
	$1^1/_2$ to $2^1/_2$	$2^1/_2$ to $3^1/_2$	$3^1/_2$ to $4^1/_2$
'Background' variables:			
social class of head of household	whether parents in receipt of benefit	highest qualification of mother	social class
highest educational qualification of child's mother			
employment status of head of household			region
region in which child living			
whether parents in receipt of Income Support or Family Credit (benefit)			whether parents in receipt of benefit
family type			
Dental care behavioural variables:			
how often mother goes to dentist	who brushes child's teeth	age started toothbrushing	frequency of toothbrushing
whether child has been seen/ examined by dentist			
age child started toothbrushing			age started toothbrushing
how often child's teeth brushed			
who brushes child's teeth			how often mother goes to dentist
Dietary behavioural variables:			
whether child ever used bottle	whether usually having drink containing sugars in bed	whether usually having drink containing sugars in bed	household spending on confectionery
whether child ever used dinky feeder			
whether child ever used dummy			
frequency of consuming sugar confectionery†		frequency of having carbonated drinks†	frequency of having carbonated drinks
frequency of consuming carbonated drinks†			
household spending on confectionery			
whether child usually having drink containing sugars in bed		household spending on confectionery	frequency of having sugar confectionery
			whether ever used a dinky feeder

* Logistic regression used with forward stepwise method. Decay experience measured as whether or not child had any experience of decay.
† Food frequency data.

Table 6.18 Variables found to be independently related to decay experience, by age

Variables put into model*	Age of child (in years)		
	1¹/₂ to 2¹/₂	2¹/₂ to 3¹/₂	3¹/₂ to 4¹/₂
social class of head of household highest educational qualification of child's mother region in which child living whether parents in receipt of Income Support or Family Credit (benefit) how often mother goes to the dentist age child started toothbrushing how often child's teeth brushed who brushes child's teeth whether child ever used dinky feeder frequency of consuming sugar confectionery† frequency of consuming carbonated drinks† household spending on confectionery whether child usually having drink containing sugars in bed	whether parents in receipt of benefit who brushes child's teeth	highest qualification of child's mother whether usually having drink containing sugars in bed	social class region household spending on confectionery whether parents in receipt of benefit

* Logistic regression used with forward stepwise method. Decay experience measured as whether or not child had any experience of decay; all variables identified as significant in Table 6.17 put into model.
† Food frequency data.

Support or Family Credit was the most significant variable identified by the model, while the highest educational qualification of children's mothers and the social class of the head of household were most significant for 2¹/₂ to 3¹/₂ and 3¹/₂ to 4¹/₂ year olds respectively.

For children aged 2¹/₂ to 3¹/₂ and 3¹/₂ to 4¹/₂ years, none of the dental care measures had an independent relationship with decay experience once the most significant background characteristic had been controlled for. For children aged 1¹/₂ to 2¹/₂ years, who brushed the child's teeth remained significant, independent of whether children's parents were in receipt of Income Support or Family Credit.

For children aged 2¹/₂ to 3¹/₂ years and 3¹/₂ to 4¹/₂ years respectively, consumption of drinks containing NME sugars

Table 6.19 The proportion of children with decay experience according to the frequency with which children were reported to consume sugar confectionery and carbonated drinks, and the frequency of toothbrushing, by age

Food frequency data

Frequency of consuming sugar confectionery and carbonated drinks and frequency of toothbrushing	Age of child (in years)							
	1¹/₂-2¹/₂		2¹/₂-3¹/₂		3¹/₂-4¹/₂		All ages	
	%*	Base	%*	Base	%*	Base	%*	Base
Sugar confectionery								
Consume more than once a day, daily or most days, and teeth brushed:								
More than once a day	6	70	17	126	33	130	21	326
Once a day	4	49	15	91	44	87	24	227
Less than once a day	[3]	28	29	34	54	37	33	99
Consume less frequently than above, or never, and teeth brushed:								
More than once a day	3	152	9	175	17	193	10	520
Once a day	2	122	12	83	32	73	13	278
Less than once a day	7	30	[5]	29	[5]	15	16	74
Carbonated drinks								
Consume more than once a day, daily or most days, and teeth brushed:								
More than once a day	[1]	28	16	64	37	74	23	166
Once a day	3	32	23	47	49	55	29	134
Less than once a day	[1]	15	30	30	[15]	28	34	73
Consume less frequently than above, or never, and teeth brushed:								
More than once a day	4	194	11	237	20	247	12	680
Once a day	2	139	10	127	32	105	14	371
Less than once a day	9	43	18	34	[10]	24	20	101

* This table shows the percentage of children with any decay experience; each percentage is calculated on the base in the right hand column. The column percentages do not total 100%.

at night and average household expenditure on confectionery were found to be related to decay experience regardless of children's backgrounds.

6.6 Relationships between dietary behaviour and dental habits and decay experience

In general the dental care variables represent behaviour designed to improve dental health while the dietary variables consider practices likely to damage the teeth. Table 6.19 groups children according to their frequency of consuming each of sugar confectionery and carbonated drinks and their frequency of toothbrushing. The proportion of children with dental decay was lowest among infrequent consumers of sugar confectionery and carbonated drinks who had their teeth brushed most often, and highest among frequent consumers of these foods and drinks who brushed their teeth least frequently. For example, 54% of $3^1/_2$ to $4^1/_2$ year olds who consumed sugar confectionery most days or more often, and who brushed their teeth less than once a day had experience of decay, compared with 17% of those who consumed sugar confectionery less frequently and brushed their teeth more than once a day (p<0.01). Overall the benefits of frequent brushing of teeth did not appear to outweigh the damaging effects of frequent sugars consumption. For example, more decay experience was found among the frequent consumers of sugar confectionery who brushed their teeth more than once a day (21%) than among the less frequent consumers who brushed their teeth less than once a day (16%) (difference not significant, p>0.05).

References and notes

[1] O'Brien M. *Children's dental health in the United Kingdom 1993*. HMSO (1994).

[2] Fluoride supplements are not nutritional supplements. The terminology is used in this Report to reflect common usage in the dental profession.

[3] Sugars may be classified as intrinsic or extrinsic:
Extrinsic sugars are not located within the cellular structure of food, they are either free in food or added to it. Extrinsic sugars are further classified as
- *milk sugars* (mainly lactose) naturally occurring in milk and milk products
- *non-milk extrinsic sugars*
Intrinsic sugars are naturally integrated into the cellular structure of a food. The most important sources are whole fruits and vegetables containing mainly fructose, glucose and sucrose.

Non-milk extrinsic sugars are considered to be particularly damaging to the teeth.[8]

[4] In the dental interview over 20 types of drinks were listed. For the purpose of analysis in this chapter, drinks have been grouped into more general categories as follows:

milk -	cow's milk, infant formula, breast milk
water -	water
drinks containing, or with added sugars -	Fruit squash with sugar, hot chocolate, Ovaltine, Horlicks, flavoured milk, tea and coffee with sugar, blackcurrant drink, fruit juice or syrup, carbonated drinks (including low calorie carbonated drinks).
other drinks, not containing sugars -	fruit squash without sugar, low calorie blackcurrant drink, tea or coffee without sugar.

[5] Readers wishing to interpret these data should refer back to Chapter 5 (section 5.7.2) for discussion of the way in which measures were calculated, and possible limitations.

[6] Gregory J R. Collins D L. Davies P S W. Hughes J M. Clarke P C. National Diet and Nutrition Survey: children aged $1^1/_2$ to $4^1/_2$ years. Volume 1: *Report of the diet and nutrition survey* HMSO (1995) (Chapter 4).

[7] Consumption and intake values at the 10th and 90th percentiles are shown in Chapter 5, Table 5.25. Although it would be expected that a tenth of the children in the survey would be included in each percentile, at the 10th percentile, the average daily consumption of sugar confectionery, chocolate confectionery, soft drinks and fruit juice, was zero for children of all ages. All the children who were non-consumers of these foods fall into the lowest consuming group, and so the bases for the lowest percentile in fact represent more than 10% of children in the survey.

[8] Department of Health *Dietary sugars and Human Disease*. London HMSO, 1989 (Reports on Health and Social Subjects:37).

[9] Variables included in the model had differences in decay experience between categories which were significant at the 95% level (p<0.05). The first variable to be selected by the model was the one which had the highest significance value. Additional variables had to meet the criteria of differences significant at the 95% level, with the effect of variables already in the model being controlled for. The logistic regression only identified relationships in priority order; the strengths of the independent associations cannot be obtained from this technique.

7 Trauma to the incisors and erosion of the upper incisors

7.1 Introduction

This chapter is divided into two parts; the first covers trauma, or accidental damage, to the incisors as recorded in the dental examination and the second considers erosion of the upper incisors, again using data from the dental examination.

7.2 Trauma to the incisors

The identification of trauma to the upper and lower incisors was the second component of the dental examination; full examinations for this component were achieved for 1570 children. The dentists recorded trauma of various types; discolouration of teeth, fractures - into the enamel, dentine and dental pulp, teeth missing due to trauma, restorations due to trauma and teeth displaced due to trauma.[1] Overall, the teeth of 15% of children aged $1^1/_2$ to $4^1/_2$ years had experienced trauma (Table 7.1). Children in the youngest age cohort were less likely to have experienced dental trauma than older children and prevalence was higher among boys than girls, although differences by age and sex did not reach statistical significance (p>0.05). Most of the trauma affected teeth on the upper jaw; 15% of children had experienced trauma to the upper incisors while only 2% had experienced trauma to the lower incisors. *(Table 7.2)*

The mean number of teeth affected by trauma was 0.2 overall. Among children with some experience of dental trauma a mean of 1.4 teeth were affected. *(Table 7.3)*

Fractures were the most common type of trauma recorded. Overall 59% of children with some dental trauma had a fracture of the enamel (that is, 9% of all children aged $1^1/_2$ to $4^1/_2$ years) and 14% had a tooth where the fracture extended into the dentine. Fractures into the pulp were rare, affecting only 2% of those whose teeth had suffered some accidental damage. Discoloured teeth affected 22% of those with some trauma and 8% had lost a tooth due to trauma. Displaced teeth were recorded for 3% of children with some trauma. *(Table 7.4)*

The proportions of children with trauma did not vary significantly by social class or region (tables not shown).

7.3 Erosion of the upper incisors

Dental erosion has been defined as the loss of dental hard tissue by a chemical process that does not involve bacteria.[2] The main causes of dental erosion are considered to be extrinsic factors associated with dietary habits; for example,

Table 7.1 Proportion of children with experience of trauma to the incisors, by sex and age

Sex of child and condition of incisors	Age of child (in years)			
	$1^1/_2$ - $2^1/_2$	$2^1/_2$ - $3^1/_2$	$3^1/_2$ - $4^1/_2$	All ages
	%	%	%	%
Boys				
Experience of trauma	13	19	18	17
No experience of trauma	87	81	82	83
Base	*241*	*293*	*274*	*808*
Girls				
Experience of trauma	9	17	15	14
No experience of trauma	91	83	85	86
Base	*233*	*263*	*266*	*762*
Boys and girls				
Experience of trauma	11	18	16	15
No experience of trauma	89	82	84	85
Base	*474*	*556*	*540*	*1570*

Table 7.2 Proportion of children with experience of trauma to the incisors in the upper and lower jaws by age

Condition of incisors	Age of child (in years)			
	$1^1/_2$ - $2^1/_2$	$2^1/_2$ - $3^1/_2$	$3^1/_2$ - $4^1/_2$	All ages
	Percentage of children with trauma			
Experience of trauma to upper incisors	10	17	15	15
Experience of trauma to lower incisors	2	1	2	2
Base	*474*	*556*	*540*	*1570*

Table 7.3 The mean number of incisors with experience of trauma for all children and children with some trauma, by age

Child group	Age of child (in years)			
	$1^1/_2$ - $2^1/_2$	$2^1/_2$ - $3^1/_2$	$3^1/_2$ - $4^1/_2$	All ages
All children	0.2	0.3	0.2	0.2
Base	*474*	*556*	*540*	*1570*
Children with some trauma	1.4	1.4	1.5	1.4
Base	*53*	*101*	*88*	*242*

Table 7.4 Types of trauma recorded for children with some trauma to the incisors, by age

Type of trauma	Age of child (in years)			
	$1^1/_2$ - $2^1/_2$	$2^1/_2$ - $3^1/_2$	$3^1/_2$ - $4^1/_2$	All ages
	*Percentage of children with each type of trauma**			
Discolouration of tooth	13	16	34	22
Fracture - into the tooth enamel only	66	67	45	59
- into the enamel and dentine	19	18	8	14
- into the dental pulp	2	1	2	2
Tooth missing due to trauma	6	5	12	8
Tooth restored after trauma	0	2	1	0
Tooth displaced by trauma	6	4	1	3
Base	*53*	*101*	*88*	*242*

* Percentages may add to more than 100% as children may have experienced more than one type of trauma.

the consumption of demineralizing acidic foods such as citric fruits and acidic beverages.[3]

While dental erosion has attracted considerable attention in the literature in recent years, the 1993 survey of school children's dental health[4] made the first attempt to assess the national prevalence of dental erosion among children aged 5 to 15 years in the United Kingdom. This survey of preschool children's dental health also included an assessment of erosion, drawing on the methodology developed for the children's dental health survey. The upper incisors were examined on both the buccal and palatal surfaces and for each surface an assessment was made as to whether there was erosion into the enamel, erosion into the dentine or erosion into the pulp. While this chapter presents the findings of these assessments, it should be noted that erosion, especially that into the enamel only, can be difficult to identify and different dentists may have made different assessments.[5] Moreover, complete examinations were more difficult to obtain for erosion than for other components of the examination; this component was at the end of the examination and the palatal surfaces could only be examined with the aid of a mirror. Findings in this section should therefore be interpreted with more caution than those for other components of the dental examination.

Complete examinations of the buccal surfaces were achieved for 1522 children and 1496 children had a complete examination for palatal erosion.

Overall, 10% of children were recorded as having any dental erosion on the buccal surfaces of their teeth and 19% were found to have erosion on the palatal surfaces (Table 7.5). Erosion into the dentine or pulp, which was least likely to be mis-identified and which may also have treatment implications, affected the buccal surfaces of the teeth of 2% of children and the palatal surfaces of 8%. The prevalence of erosion increased by age, with 3% of children aged $1^1/_2$ to $2^1/_2$ years found to have some palatal erosion into the dentine or pulp compared with 13% of those aged $3^1/_2$ to $4^1/_2$ years.

Table 7.6 shows the mean numbers of teeth with erosion for all children in the sample, and for those who were recorded as having some erosion. Overall, children were recorded as

having 0.3 teeth with buccal erosion and 0.6 teeth with palatal erosion. The mean numbers of teeth with erosion into the dentine or pulp were 0.1 and 0.2 for buccal and palatal surfaces respectively. Children who were recorded as having some erosion, were generally found to have most of the four teeth examined, affected. Thus an average of 3.2 teeth were recorded as having erosion on both the buccal and palatal surfaces among those where some erosion was reported on these surfaces. Among children with palatal surface erosion into dentine or pulp a mean of 2.7 teeth were affected. Among children with some erosion the mean number of teeth affected did not vary significantly by age.

The distribution of erosion between the incisors is shown in Table 7.7. Data relating only to the left side of the mouth are shown as the pattern on the left and right sides was found to be very similar. For each age group the proportion of children with eroded central incisors was virtually the same as the proportion with any erosion shown in Table 7.5. The lateral incisors were affected among a smaller proportion of children, especially on the palatal surfaces. For example, among $3^1/_2$ to $4^1/_2$ year olds 12% of children had palatal erosion into the dentine or pulp on their central incisor compared with 5% having such erosion on their lateral incisor. On the buccal surfaces, 3% had erosion into the dentine or pulp on both their central and lateral incisors.

Table 7.5 Proportion of children with any erosion recorded on buccal and palatal surfaces of incisors and with any erosion into dentine or pulp, by age

Condition of incisors	Age of child (in years)			
	$1^1/_2$ - $2^1/_2$	$2^1/_2$ - $3^1/_2$	$3^1/_2$ - $4^1/_2$	All ages
	Percentage of children with erosion			
Buccal surfaces				
any erosion	7	10	14	10
erosion into dentine or pulp	1	2	3	2
Base	*462*	*545*	*515*	*1522*
Palatal surfaces				
any erosion	9	18	29	19
erosion into dentine or pulp	3	6	13	8
Base	*445*	*533*	*518*	*1496*

Table 7.6 The mean number of teeth with any erosion and erosion into the dentine or pulp for buccal and palatal surfaces; means shown for all children and for children with some erosion of type specified, by age

Child group and type of erosion	Age of child (in years)			
	$1^1/_2$ - $2^1/_2$	$2^1/_2$ - $3^1/_2$	$3^1/_2$ - $4^1/_2$	All ages
All children				
Any buccal erosion	0.3	0.3	0.4	0.3
Buccal erosion into dentine or pulp	0	0.1	0.1	0.1
Base	*462*	*545*	*515*	*1522*
Any palatal erosion	0.3	0.6	0.9	0.6
Palatal erosion into dentine or pulp	0.1	0.2	0.3	0.2
Base	*445*	*533*	*518*	*1496*
Children with some erosion				
Any buccal erosion	3.5	3.2	3.1	3.2
Base	*33*	*54*	*72*	*159*
Buccal erosion into dentine or pulp	[2.8]	[2.3]	[2.3]	2.4
Base	*6*	*12*	*15*	*33*
Any palatal erosion	3.3	3.2	3.1	3.2
Base	*42*	*98*	*154*	*294*
Palatal erosion into dentine or pulp	[3.1]	2.7	3.1	2.7
Base	*14*	*33*	*68*	*115*

53

Table 7.7 Proportion of children with erosion on individual deciduous teeth by age

Surface of tooth	Age of child (in years)			
	1½ - 2½	2½ - 3½	3½ - 4½	All ages
	Percentage of children with erosion			
Buccal surface				
central incisor				
any erosion	7	9	13	9
erosion into dentine or pulp	1	2	3	2
lateral incisor				
any erosion	6	6	12	7
erosion into dentine or pulp	0	1	3	1
Base	*462*	*545*	*515*	*1522*
Palatal surface				
central incisor				
any erosion	9	17	28	19
erosion into dentine or pulp	3	5	12	7
lateral incisor				
any erosion	7	12	17	12
erosion into dentine or pulp	2	3	5	3
Base	*445*	*533*	*518*	*1496*

Table 7.8 Area of the tooth surface affected by erosion on eroded teeth

Extent of surface covered by erosion	Age of child (in years)			
	1½ - 2½	2½ - 3½	3½ - 4½	All ages
	%	%	%	%
Buccal surface of				
central incisor				
Less than a third	27	16	31	25
A third, but less than two thirds	24	25	25	25
Two thirds or more	49	59	42	50
Base	*33*	*51*	*64*	*148*
Buccal surface of				
lateral incisor				
Less than a third	[7]	18	28	25
A third, but less than two thirds	[7]	21	23	24
Two thirds or more	[13]	61	45	51
Base	*27*	*33*	*47*	*107*
Palatal suface of				
central incisor				
Less than a third	17	18	21	20
A third, but less than two thirds	27	25	30	28
Two thirds or more	56	57	48	52
Base	*41*	*92*	*145*	*278*
Palatial surface of				
lateral incisor				
Less than a third	[5]	15	20	18
A third, but less than two thirds	[10]	17	24	23
Two thirds or more	[14]	68	56	59
Base	*29*	*66*	*91*	*186*

Dentists were also asked to assess how much of the surface area of the tooth was covered by any erosion they had identified. In 50% of cases where buccal erosion was recorded on the central or lateral incisors, two thirds or more of the tooth surface was said to be affected; for 25% of cases the erosion covered less than a third of the tooth and in the remaining 25% of cases between a third and two thirds of the surface was said to be eroded. For palatal erosion, a slightly higher proportion of children were found to have erosion extending over a third or more of the surface for both the central and lateral incisors (80% and 82% respectively). The area of the tooth surface recorded as being affected by erosion did not vary for children of different ages. *(Table 7.8)*

This Report includes no commentary comparing erosion for children with different background and behavioural characteristics. This is due to the small bases for children with erosion into the dentine or pulp, and the variability suspected between dentists' assessments for erosion into the enamel.

Tables relating erosion to some of the measures that were related to caries experience in earlier chapters are shown in Appendix E. Significant relationships between erosion and background characteristics, dental care and dietary behaviour were not found.

References and notes

[1] See Appendix A of this Report for the dentists' written instructions describing how codes should be allocated to conditions.

[2] Pindborg J J (1970) *Pathology of Dental Hard Tissues*, Copenhagen: Munksgaard, pp 312-321.

[3] Jarvinen V K Rytomaa I I Heinonen (1991) Risk Factors in Dental Erosion, *J Dent Res 70(6) pp942-947*.

[4] O'Brien M. *Children's dental health in the United Kingdom 1993* HMSO (1994).

[5] The training of dentists for the school and preschool children's dental health surveys differed; dentists working on the former survey attended a two day residential course while those working on the less complicated preschool children's survey attended only a one day briefing and had less detailed written instructions.[1] The training for the schoolchildren's survey included a calibration exercise designed to assess the degree of similarity in the way dentists recorded different conditions. Evidence from this calibration exercise indicated that dentists found it difficult to agree in determining the presence of erosion of the enamel. Further information is contained in Appendix F of the report of the 1993 children's dental health survey.[4]

Appendices

Appendix A Dentists' criteria for the dental examination

The examination procedure

There is no set procedure for the dental examination in this study. We would suggest that the child is placed in whatever position is thought to be the most suitable, as dictated by each individual occasion. Some examiners find it easiest to look at children of this age with them lying on the floor, however, that is only a suggestion.

There will be no standard light source prescribed for this study. We would suggest that you get each child in the best light available and supplement this with a pen torch if necessary.

The only equipment necessary for each examination will be a small mirror. The survey does not require the use of probes for diagnosis. If you wish to have a blunt probe available to remove gross debris, then please do so, however should you prefer to use cotton wool rolls, gauze etc for removing gross debris, then please use that method.

We would remind each examiner that they should use a fresh pair of gloves for each child and a freshly sterilised probe and any other instruments or material they might use for removing debris. White coats will obviously not be necessary.

As background information, all the children you see will have been part of a larger dietary study. This will have involved their parents in keeping a record of their diet over a period of four days and weighing and measuring everything they eat. In addition, I understand that some time during their period of contact with OPCS, each child for whom permission has been given will have a blood sample taken by a local phlebotomist.

Some children may well be very difficult to examine, it is left to your best judgement to decide whether to complete the examination when the circumstances become difficult.

THE STATE OF THE TEETH

A diagnosis of the state of each tooth will be made and recorded using the codes shown below:

Code 0   The tooth is present in the mouth and is not carious, filled or traumatised. A tooth is considered sound if any part of that tooth is present in the mouth.

Code 1   Teeth are regarded as traumatised if they are not decayed and show evidence of damage due to trauma. If they contain a temporary or permanent restoration following trauma, they are included in this category. Teeth are also included in this category if they are absent from the mouth as a result of traumatic damage.

Code 2   Teeth will be recorded as decayed, if, in the opinion of the examiner, after visual examination, any surface has a carious cavity which extends into dentine, but not as extensive as code 3. Lesions containing a temporary dressing or cavities from which a restoration had been lost are included in this category.

Code 3   Teeth will be recorded in this category, if, on visual examination, it contains a carious cavity that extends into the pulp. When two-thirds or more of the marginal ridge of a deciduous molar is carious, it is included in this category.

Code 4   The tooth contains a permanent restoration of any material and no carious cavities which could be classified in code 2 & 3. Teeth containing a permanent restoration and a carious cavity are coded as 2 or 3, whichever is appropriate.

Code 5   Teeth will be regarded as missing if they have been extracted because it was carious. Teeth which are absent for any other reason are not included in the category. If roots were seen to be remaining, the tooth is recorded as decayed, with pulpal involvement.

Code 6   Teeth are regarded as unerupted if they had not erupted into the mouth, that is, no part of the tooth was visible.

If doubt exists, the lower or better category is scored. Blunt probes are used, only for the removal of gross food deposits obscuring the tooth surfaces. No measure of dental cleanliness will be used in this study.

TRAUMA OF PRIMARY INCISORS

Upper and lower incisors will be examined for traumatic injury and recorded as follows:

Code 1   Discolouration
Code 2   Fracture involving enamel
Code 3   Fracture involving enamel and dentine
Code 4   Fracture involving enamel, dentine and pulp
Code 5   Missing due to trauma
Code 6   Restoration such as glass ionomer, composite or stainless steel crown
Code 7   Incisor displaced by trauma

EROSION OF INCISORS

The labial surfaces of primary maxillary incisor teeth will be assessed for loss of surface enamel characteristics, and/or exposure of dentine or pulp.

DO NOT consider the incisal edge.

Assess the **Depth** and **Area** of loss of tooth tissue for each surface using the following criteria:

Depth

Code 0	Normal
Code 1	Enamel only - loss of surface characterisation.
Code 2	Enamel and Dentine - loss of enamel, exposing dentine.
Code 3	Enamel into Pulp - loss of enamel and dentine resulting in pulpal exposure.

Area

For each affected surface assess by area:

Code 1	Less than one third of surface involved.
Code 2	One third - up to two thirds of surface involved.
Code 3	More than two thirds of surface involved.

CHILD'S CO-OPERATION

Grade 1
Easy Examination

A full visual oral examination was achieved with no difficulty. The child responded immediately to the request to open their mouth. No/minimum escort was required.

Grade 2
Examination with a slight difficulty

A full visual oral examination was achieved with slight difficulty. The child responded within five minutes to the request to open their mouth. Some escort assistance (encouragement) was required. Some limitation of mouth opening may have been noted.

Grade 3
Examination with moderate difficulty

A full visual oral examination was achieved with moderate difficulty. The child took five minutes to respond to the request to open their mouth. Escort assistance was required to complete the examination. The child cried.

Grade 4
No examination possible

The child was sufficiently unco-operative not to allow any oral examination.

(From Galuszka 1990)

Appendix B Fieldwork documents

Contents

Dental recall sheet
Dental survey purpose leaflet
Dental Survey questionnaire
Dental show cards
Dietary survey interview schedule
Dietary survey show cards
Instructions and sample page of 4-day weighed intake diary
Full fieldwork documents for the dietary survey, including advance letters included in the Report of the dietary survey.[1]

[1] Gregory JR Collins DL Davies PSW Hughes JM Clarke PC. *National Diet and Nutrition Survey: children aged 1¹/₂ to 4¹/₂ years.*
 Volume 1: Report of the diet and nutrition survey, HMSO (1995).

Dental recall sheet

T

Serial no. label

N1340/W4

DENTAL RECALL SHEET

Interviewer
Auth No

Today's Date: DAY MONTH YEAR
                                    9 3

Interviewer's
name

1. Ask mother or mother figure
INTRODUCE DENTAL FOLLOW UP

I would like to come back in a few weeks time to ask you some questions about your child's
dental habits. I would also like to bring a dentist with me to carry out a short examination
of his/her teeth.
Would it be alright it I called on you again ?

CODE

Yes, (agreed to interview and examination) .... 1 → (i)

Yes, (agreed to interview only) .... 2 → (i)

Yes, other/conditional .... 3 → (i)

No, unconditional .... 4 → 5

(i) May I contact you   Yes 1   TEL NO ....
by telephone if necessary ?   No 2

2. If coded 1, 2 or 3 at Q1, enter informant's name, and toddler's name and date of birth.
Copy per. no from household box.

MOTHER/ MOTHER FIGURE

PER NO   MRS/MISS/MR   INITIALS   SURNAME

CHILD

FIRST NAME   SURNAME   (Date of birth)
                                              DAY MONTH YEAR

3. Does address differ   CODE   **4. Is the child or the**   CODE
in any way from   Yes.........1   informant moving in   Yes.........1
address list ?   No 2   the next 4 months ?   No 2

If yes, give full details   If yes, give address and approx
below   date of move below

.   ...

5. IF Q1 IS CODED 2, 3, OR 4, RECORD COMMENTS

OPCS
OFFICE OF POPULATION
CENSUSES & SURVEYS

The
Young Children's
Dental Health
Survey

This survey is being carried out by the Social Survey Division of the Office of Population Censuses and Surveys for the Departments of Health (in England, Wales and Scotland). This leaflet tells you more about why the survey is being done.

• What is it about?

The Departments of Health are responsible for a wide range of services and activities to look after our teeth. In order to do this they require up-to-date, reliable information about all age-groups.

Although we know a lot about older children's teeth, little is known at a national level about the dental condition of children aged 1½ to 4½ years. For example, what proportion of these children have dental decay, and at what age does teeth brushing start?

The Departments of Health have asked Social Survey Division to carry out this dental survey of young children. They would like to find out about the dental condition and dental habits of children in this age-group and to learn more about the relationship between their diets and their dental health.

• Why have we come to your household?

To call at every address in the country would take too long and cost too much. Earlier this year, we selected a sample of addresses from the Postcode Address File and we visited your household by chance as part of the Young Children's Dietary Survey.

At that time, somebody in your household said that you might be prepared to take part in this dental survey. We have therefore come back to your household to find out if you are still prepared to take part.

• Is the survey confidential?

Yes. Any information you give will be treated in confidence. No identifiable information about you or your household will be passed to other organisations or government departments without your consent. The results will not be presented in any way in which they can be associated with your name or address. No information about you or your household will be passed to local authorities, members of the public or the press.

Dental survey purpose leaflet - *continued*

- ● *Is the survey compulsory?*

In all our surveys we rely on voluntary co-operation, which is essential if our work is to be successful.

- ● *What does it involve?*

We would like our interviewer to carry out a short interview with a parent or guardian of your child. This will take about twenty minutes.

In addition, we would like to carry out a brief examination of your child's teeth. If you agree, the examination will be carried out in your home, and at a time to suit you, by a community dentist experienced in dealing with children. It will be painless and will simply involve looking at and counting your child's teeth. The examination will take about five minutes.

We hope this leaflet answers some of the questions you might have and shows the importance of the survey.

Your co-operation is very much appreciated.

Social Survey Division
Office of Population Censuses and Surveys
St Catherine's House
10 Kingsway
London
WC2B 6JP

Telephone: 071 396 2457/2079

HA22/1 2/93

N1351 Young Children's Dental Health Survey

Dental survey interview questionnaire

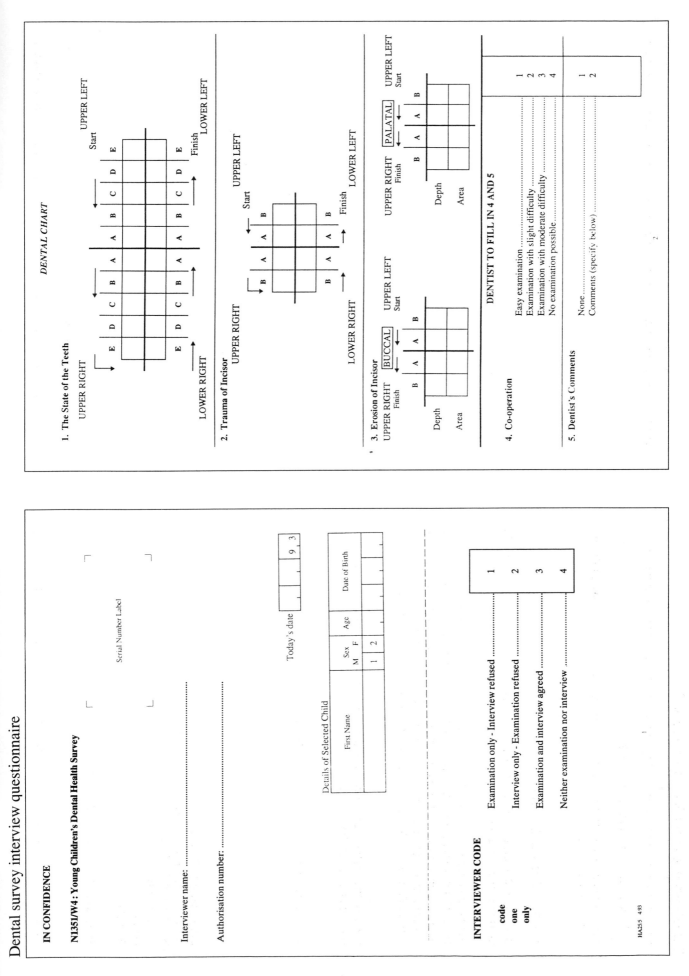

DENTAL CHART

1. The State of the Teeth

UPPER LEFT

UPPER RIGHT

Start

LOWER LEFT

Finish

LOWER RIGHT

2. Trauma of Incisor

UPPER RIGHT

UPPER LEFT

Start

LOWER RIGHT

LOWER LEFT

Finish

3. Erosion of Incisor

UPPER RIGHT
Finish

UPPER LEFT
Start

BUCCAL

UPPER RIGHT
Finish

UPPER LEFT
Start

PALATAL

Depth

Area

Depth

Area

DENTIST TO FILL IN 4 AND 5

4. Co-operation

Easy examination 1
Examination with slight difficulty 2
Examination with moderate difficulty 3
No examination possible 4

5. Dentist's Comments

None 1
Comments (specify below) 2

IN CONFIDENCE

N135IJ/W4 : Young Children's Dental Health Survey

Serial Number Label

Interviewer name: ....

Authorisation number: ....

Today's date

| | 9 | 3 |

Details of Selected Child

First Name	Sex	Age	Date of Birth
	M	F		
	1	2		

INTERVIEWER CODE

code
one
only

Examination only - Interview refused 1

Interview only - Examination refused 2

Examination and interview agreed 3

Neither examination nor interview 4

HA255 4 93

61

Dental survey interview questionnaire - *continued*

INTERVIEWER CODE

1. The State of the Teeth

Examination completed	1
Partial examination	2
Not carried out	3

2. Trauma of Incisor

Examination completed	1
Partial examination	2
Not carried out	3

3. Erosion of Incisor

Examination completed	1
Partial examination	2
Not carried out	3

INTERVIEWER CODE

(a) Who is being interviewed as informant?

Code one only

Child's mother (female parent-figure)	1
Child's father (male parent-figure)	2
Child's 'mother' and 'father' jointly	3

Enter Start Time (24 hr clock)

Hrs	Mins

DENTAL HISTORY

1. Has ...... (**CHILD**) ever been seen by a dentist apart from today, for treatment, a check-up or just to get used to going?

Yes	1
No	2

2. Is ...... (**CHILD**) registered with a dentist?

Yes	1
No	2
Don't know	3

3. May I check, has ...... (**CHILD**) actually been examined by a dentist?

No, never examined by a dentist	1	Q8
Yes, seen and examined by a dentist	2	Q4
Seen but not examined by a dentist	3	
Spontaneous only Seen by a dentist but child refused to co-operate	4	Q9

4. When was the last time ...... (**CHILD**) was seen by a dentist?

Prompt as necessary

More than 6 months ago	1
6 months ago, or more recently	2
Cannot remember	3

5. Was the last visit for:

Running prompt

treatment	1
a check-up	2
or just to get used to going?	3

6. May I check, was ...... (**CHILD**) actually examined by a dentist on that occasion?

Yes, seen and examined by a dentist	1
Seen but not examined by a dentist	2
Spontaneous only Seen by a dentist but child refused to co-operate	3

Dental survey interview questionnaire - *continued*

7. (Can I check) has ..... (CHILD) ever had:

	Yes	No	Don't know
any teeth filled?	1	2	3
any teeth taken out?	1	2	3
Individual prompt any treatment to stop teeth decaying or going bad eg by painting and/or sealing the teeth?	1	2	3
his/her teeth cleaned at the dentist?	1	2	3
any other treatment? (specify)	1	2	3
.....	1	2	3
.....	1	2	3

DNA, no teeth taken out ..... X ------- Q9

(a) IF CHILD HAS HAD TEETH TAKEN OUT

Has ..... (**CHILD**) ever had a general anaesthetic when **having teeth extracted?**

Yes	1	
No	2	} Q9
Don't know	3	

8. Have you **ever** tried to make a dental appointment for ..... (**CHILD**)?

| Yes ..... | 1 | Q9 |
| No ..... | 2 | Q10 |

9. Have you **ever** had any difficulties trying to make a dental appointment for ..... (**CHILD**)?

| Yes ..... | 1 | (a) |
| No ..... | 2 | Q10 |

(a) What sort of difficulties have you had?

[*]

10. Compared with other children, do you think ..... (CHILD) has had:

Running prompt

no difficulty teething	1
little difficulty teething	2
some difficulty teething	3
or a lot of difficulty teething?	4

11. To help ...... (**CHILD**) while teething, has he/she ever had:

	Yes	No
Individual prompt a teething ring?	1	2
balm or gel?	1	2
special teething biscuits or special rusks?	1	2
medicine or painkillers of any kind?	1	2
alcohol of any kind?	1	2
anything else? (**specify**)	1	2
.....	1	2

12. (Apart from when he/she was teething), has ...... (**CHILD**) ever had toothache?

Yes	1
No	2
Don't know	3

Blank Page

13. Have you ever had advice about what
...... (CHILD) should or should not be
eating and drinking to look after his/her teeth?

Yes	1 — (a)
No	2 — Q14

(a) Where did you get this advice from?

enter code in grid opposite

14. Have you ever had any advice about
cleaning ...... (CHILD'S) teeth?

Yes	1 — (a)
No	2 — Q15

(a) Where did you get this advice from?

enter code in grid opposite

15. Have you ever been advised to give
...... (CHILD) fluoride drops or tablets?

Yes	1 — (a)
No	2 — Q16

(a) Where did you get this advice from?

enter code in grid opposite

16. Have you ever been advised not to give
...... (CHILD) fluoride drops or tablets?

Yes	1 — (a)
No	2 — Q17

(a) Where did you get this advice from?

enter code in grid opposite

Dental survey interview questionnaire - *continued*

	Q13 (a) Advice about food	Q14 (a) Advice about cleaning teeth	Q15 (a) Advice to give fluoride	Q16 (a) Advice not to give fluoride
Dentist	01	01	01	01
Doctor	02	02	02	02
Health Visitor to the home	03	03	03	03
Dental nurse/hygienist/therapist/assistant	04	04	04	04
Child Health Clinic	05	05	05	05
Dietitian	06	06	06	06
Friend	07	07	07	07
Chemist or other shop	08	08	08	08
Relative	09	09	09	09
Books/magazines	10	10	10	10
Leaflets (eg from a health centre)	11	11	11	11
Television	12	12	12	12
Other (specify)	13	13	13	13

Code all that apply

9

17. Have you ever given ...... (CHILD) fluoride drops or tablets?

Yes .... 1 — Q18

No .... 2 — Q19

18. How old was ...... (CHILD) when he/she first started taking fluoride drops or tablets?

Under 6 months 1

6 months - under 1 year 2

1 year - under 2 years 3

2 years or over 4

Cannot remember 5

10

Dental survey interview questionnaire - *continued*

BEDTIME ROUTINE

Introduce **Bedtime Routine**

19. Who usually puts ...... (**CHILD**) to bed?

Mother (figure)	1
Father (figure)	2
Child him/herself	3
Varies	4
Other (**do not specify**)	5

20. Many children take a drink to bed with them either to have before they go to sleep, or during the night.

Nowadays how often does ...... (**CHILD**) have something to drink in bed or during the night?

Show Card A

Every night	1	→ Q21
4 - 6 nights a week	2	
1 - 3 nights a week	3	
Less often than once a week	4	
Never	5	→ Q23

---

21. When ...... (**CHILD**) has a drink in bed or during the night, what does he/she usually have?

a: Milk drinks

Cows' milk (not flavoured)	01
Infant formula	02
Breast Milk	03
Hot chocolate, Ovaltine, Horlicks, flavoured milk	04

Code all that apply

b: Fruit juices & squashes

Fruit squash/drink, contains sugar	05
Fruit squash/drink, does not contain sugar	06
Fruit juice (undiluted)	07
Fruit juice (diluted)	08
Fruit syrup (diluted)	09

c: Blackcurrant drinks

Blackcurrant drink	10
Blackcurrant drink (diet)	11

d: Fizzy drinks

Fizzy drink	12
Fizzy drink (diet)	13

Show card B

e: Tea/coffee

Tea/coffee with sugar	14
Tea/coffee without sugar	15

f: Water

Sweetened water	16
Water	17

g: Herbal drinks/tea

Herbal drink/tea, contains sugar	18
Herbal drink/tea, does not contain sugar	19

h: Other (please specify)

Other drink, contains sugar (specify)	20
Other drink, does not contain sugar (specify)	21

(a) **If more than one drink specified**

DNA, one drink only	X	→ Q22

Which of those you mentioned does he/she have most often?

enter code from list |___|

22. When ...... (**CHILD**) has a drink in **bed** or during the night, does he/she **usually** drink from:

Running prompt

a feeder beaker/beaker with a spout	1
a mug, cup or glass	2
a mug, cup or glass via a straw	3
a bottle	4
a dinky feeder	5
or from something else? (specify)	6

Code one only

Dental survey interview questionnaire - *continued*

23. Thinking about food, nowadays how often does ..... **(CHILD)** have something to eat in bed or during the night?

Show card A

Every night	1
4 - 6 nights a week	2 — Q24
1 - 3 nights a week	3
Less often than once a week	4
Never	5 — Q25

24. When ..... **(CHILD)** does have something to eat in bed or during the night, what does he/she usually have?

Code all that apply

Sweet biscuits (including chocolate biscuits)	01
Savoury and plain biscuits (including cheese biscuits)	02
Cakes	03
Crisps or savoury snacks	04
Fruit	05
Sandwiches (sweet)	06
Sandwiches (savoury)	07
Sweets or chocolate	08
Other (specify)	09

(a) If more than one food item specified

DNA, one food item only	X — Q25
Which of those you mentioned does he/she have most often? enter code from list	:.....:

13

Introduce

25. (Opinions vary as to at what age children should start brushing their teeth. Also, some children refuse to have anything to do with it until they are quite old.)

Has ..... **(CHILD)** started brushing his/her teeth or having his/her teeth brushed?

Yes	1 — Q26
No	2 — Q37

26. How old was ..... **(CHILD)** when he/she first started having his/her teeth brushed?

Under 1 year	1
1 year - under 2 years	2
2 years - under 3 years	3
3 years or over	4
Cannot remember	5

27. (As well as children objecting to it, there are different opinions as to how often children should have their teeth brushed.)

So on the whole, how often does ..... **(CHILD)** brush his/her teeth or have them brushed?

Show card C

Less often than once a week	1
At least once a week but not every day	2
Once a day	3
More than once a day	4

28. At what time(s) of day are ..... **(CHILD'S)** teeth usually brushed?

Code all that apply

Prompt as necessary

Before breakfast	1
Just after breakfast	2
At bedtime, but might eat or drink something afterwards	3
At bedtime, but after all eating is finished	4
Just after other meal(s) [not breakfast/not at bedtime]	5
At other times	6
Varies	7

Dental survey interview questionnaire - *continued*

29. (Some children insist on brushing their own teeth from a very early age.)

Does ...... (CHILD): brush his/her own teeth ...... 1 — Q30

Running prompt does he/she have it done for him/her ...... 2 — Q31

or does he/she sometimes do it alone and sometimes have it done for him/her? 3

If an adult always assists or repeats = 2

30. How old was ......(CHILD) when he/she started cleaning his/her teeth on his/her own?

Under 2 years 1

2 years - under 3 years 2

3 years or over 3

Cannot remember ...... 4 — (a)

(a) Has ...... (CHILD) always cleaned his/her own teeth?

Yes 1

No, someone else used to help 2

31. (People start using toothpaste at different ages.)

Has ...... (CHILD) started using toothpaste?

Yes ...... 1 — (a)

No ...... 2 — Q34

(a) How old was ...... (CHILD) when you first used toothpaste for him/her?

Under 1 year 1

1 year - under 2 years 2

2 years - under 3 years 3

3 years or over 4

Cannot remember 5

32. Nowadays, when ...... (CHILD'S) teeth are brushed, is it:

sometimes with toothpaste 1

Running prompt often with toothpaste 2

or always with toothpaste? 3

33. What brand of toothpaste does ...... (CHILD) use at the moment?

Record brand name (main one if there is more than one)

....

34. Families sometimes share a toothbrush; At present:

Running prompt is ...... (CHILD) sharing a toothbrush with anyone else 1

or does he/she have his/her own? 2

35. What size is the toothbrush that ...... (CHILD) usually uses; is it:

Running prompt an adult 1

or a junior, or a very small toothbrush? 2

36. DNA, has not started using toothpaste (Q31 coded 2) ...... X ----- Q37

How much toothpaste does ...... (CHILD) usually use on his/her toothbrush; does it cover:

Running prompt most or all of the brush 1

or just a small part of the brush? 2

Spontaneous only about half the length of the brush 3

BOTTLE, DINKY FEEDER AND DUMMY

37. (You may have told me about this already, but may I check) has ..... (CHILD) <u>ever used</u>:

	Yes	No	
a bottle, even just to go to bed with?	1	2	–if 2 (no bottle); ring DNA column A below
INCLUDE BOTTLES CONTAINING DRINKS OTHER THAN MILK/FORMULA			
Individual prompt — a dinky feeder?	1	2	–if 2 (no dinky feeder); ring DNA column B below
a dummy?	1	2	–if 2 (no dummy); ring DNA column C below

COMPLETE COLUMN A (IF APPLIES) UNTIL THE END OF THE COLUMN ON PAGE 19 OR PAGE 21

THEN COMPLETE COLUMN B (IF APPLIES) UNTIL THE END OF THE COLUMN ON PAGE 19 OR 21

THEN COMPLETE COLUMN C

38. How old was ..... (CHILD) when he/she first used a _____?

	A Bottle	B Dinky Feeder	C Dummy
DNA......	X → col B	X → col C	...X → Q48 p23
Under 6 months	1	1	1
6 months - under 1 year	2	2	2
1 year - under 2 years	3	3	3
2 years - under 3 years	4	4	4
3 years or over	5	5	5
Cannot remember	6	6	6

39. (May I check) these days, does ..... (CHILD) use a _____ at all (even just to go to bed with)?

	A Bottle	B Dinky Feeder	C Dummy
Yes	1 → Q41	1 → Q41	1 → Q41
No	2 → Q40	2 → Q40	2 → Q40

40. How old was ..... (CHILD) when he/she stopped using a _____?

	A Bottle	B Dinky Feeder	C Dummy
Under 6 months	1	1	1
6 months - under 1 year	2	2	2
1 year - under 2 years	3 – Q44	3 – Q44	3 – Q44
2 years - under 3 years......	4	4	4
3 years or over	5	5	5
Cannot remember	6	6	6

41. These days, in bed or during the night, how often does ..... (CHILD) use a _____?

Show Card A

	A Bottle	B Dinky Feeder	C Dummy
Every night	1	1	1
4 - 6 nights a week	2	2	2
1 - 3 nights a week	3 – Q42	3 – Q42	3 – Q47
Less often than once a week	4	4	4
Never, only during the day	5	5	5

42. Apart from in bed or during the night, how often does ..... (CHILD) use a _____?

	A Bottle	B Dinky Feeder	C Dummy
Never, only at night	1	1	
Less often than once a day	2	2	
Once a day	3	3	
Twice a day	4	4	
3 times a day	5	5	
4 times or more a day	6	6	

Dental survey interview questionnaire - *continued*

Q43

	A Bottle	B Dinky Feeder	C Dummy

43. Which of the following does he/she have in his/her _____ during the day or at night?

		A Bottle	B Dinky Feeder
a: Milk drinks	Cows' milk (not flavoured)	01	01
	Infant formula	02	02
	Breast Milk	03	03
	Hot chocolate, Ovaltine, Horlicks, flavoured milk	04	04
b: Fruit juices & squashes (Show Card B)	Fruit squash/drink, contains sugar	05	05
	Fruit squash/drink, does not contain sugar	06	06
	Fruit juice (undiluted)	07	07
	Fruit juice (diluted)	08	08
	Fruit syrup (diluted)	09	09
c: Blackcurrant drinks	Blackcurrant drink, contains sugar	10	10
	Blackcurrant drink (diet)	11	11
d: Fizzy drinks	Fizzy drink	12 (a)	12 (a)
	Fizzy drink (diet)	13	13
e: Tea/coffee	Tea/coffee with sugar	14	14
	Tea/coffee without sugar	15	15
f: Water	Sweetened water	16	16
	Water	17	17
g: Herbal drinks/tea	Herbal drink/tea, contains sugar	18	18
	Herbal drink/tea, does not contain sugar	19	19
h: Other (please specify)	Other drink, contains sugar (specify)	20	20
	Other drink, does not contain sugar (specify)	21	21

If more than one drink specified ask (a) and (b)

DNA, one drink only ...... X → see Q38 col B | X → see Q38 col C

(a) Ask of all who have a _____ in bed or at night

DNA if no _____ in bed or at night (Q41 coded 5)....X→ (b) | ...X → (b)

Which of those drinks does he/she have most often in his/her _____ in bed or during the night?

enter code from list | enter code from list

(b) Ask all of who have a _____ at other times of day

DNA if no _____ at other times of day (Q42 coded 1)...X→ see Q38 col B | .X→ see Q38 col C

Apart from in bed or during the night) Which of those drinks does he/she have most often in his/her _____?

enter code from list see Q38 col B | enter code from list see Q38 col C

19

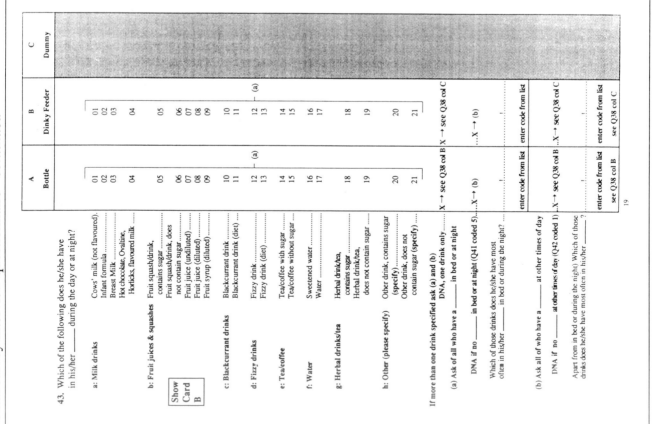

	A Bottle	B Dinky Feeder	C Dummy

44. Just before ...... (CHILD) stopped using a _____, how often did he/she have one in bed or during the night?

Show Card A

	A Bottle	B Dinky Feeder	C Dummy
Every night	1	1	1
4 - 6 nights a week	2	2	2
1 - 3 nights a week	3 ─Q45	3 ─Q45	3 ─Q47
Less often than once a week	4	4	4
Never, only during the day	5	5	5

45. Apart from in bed or during the night, just before ...... (CHILD) stopped using a _____, how often did he/she have one?

	A Bottle	B Dinky Feeder
Never, only at night	1	1
Less often than once a day	2	2
Once a day	3	3
Twice a day	4	4
3 times a day	5	5
4 times or more a day	6	6

20

Dental survey interview questionnaire - *continued*

46. Just before ...... **(CHILD)** stopped using a _____, which of the following did he/she <u>have in it during the day or night?</u>

Show Card B

		A Bottle	B Dinky Feeder	C Dummy
a: Milk drinks	Cows' milk (not flavoured)	01	01	
	Infant formula	02	02	
	Breast Milk	03	03	
	Hot chocolate, Ovaltine, Horlicks, flavoured milk	04	04	
b: Fruit juices & squashes	Fruit squash/drink, contains sugar	05	05	
	Fruit squash/drink, does not contain sugar	06	06	
	Fruit juice (undiluted)	07	07	
	Fruit juice (diluted)	08	08	
	Fruit syrup (diluted)	09	09	
c: Blackcurrant drinks	Blackcurrant drink	10	10	
	Blackcurrant drink (diet)	11	11	
d: Fizzy drinks	Fizzy drink	12 (a)	12 (a)	
	Fizzy drink (diet)	13	13	
e: Tea/coffee	Tea/coffee with sugar	14	14	
	Tea/coffee without sugar	15	15	
f: Water	Sweetened water	16	16	
	Water	17	17	
g: Herbal drinks/tea	Herbal drink/tea, contains sugar	18	18	
	Herbal drink/tea, does not contain sugar	19	19	
h: Other (please specify)	Other drink, contains sugar (specify)	20	20	
	Other drink, does not contain sugar (specify)	21	21	

If more than one drink specified ask (a) and (b)

(a) Ask all of who had a _____ in bed or at night

DNA, one drink only ...... X → see Q38 col B ...X → see Q38 col C

DNA if no _____ in bed or at night (Q44 coded 5) ...X → (b) ...X → (b)

Which of those drinks does he/she have most often in his/her _____ in bed or during the night?

enter code from list | enter code from list

(b) Ask all of who had a _____ at other times of day

DNA if no _____ at other times of day (Q45 coded 1) ...X → see Q38 col B ...X → see Q38 col C

(Apart from in bed or during the night) Which of those drinks did he/she have most often in his/her _____ ?

enter code from list | enter code from list

see Q38 col B | see Q38 col C

21

---

47. To make the dummy taste nice, has it ever been dipped into anything sweet?

Yes .... 1 → (a)

No .... 2 → Q48

(a) What was it dipped into?

Honey 1

Jam 2

Other (specify) 3

22

Dental survey interview questionnaire - continued

CONFECTIONERY

Introduce

48. How old was ..... (CHILD) when he/she first tasted

Individual prompt

(a) chocolate?

(b) other sweets?

(c) sweet biscuits?

record in grid below

	(a) chocolate	(b) other sweets	(c) sweet biscuits
Under 6 months	1	1	1
6 months - under 1 year	2	2	2
1 year - under 2 years	3	3	3
2 years or over	4	4	4
Never	5	5	5
Cannot remember/don't know	6	6	6

49. On average, how much does your household spend on chocolates and sweets a week:

nothing 1

less than two pounds a week 2

Running prompt   between two and five pounds a week 3

or more than five pounds a week? 4

(Don't know) 5

50. Does **anybody** else give sweets or chocolates to ......(CHILD) at least once a week?

Yes .... 1 ──(a)

No .... 2 ──Q51

Don't know 3

(a) **Who** would this be?

Grandparent 1

Other (specify) 2

23

Introduce

51. **Applies if informant is child's mother (female parent-figure)**

or if informant is child's father (male parent-figure) AND no "mother" in household

DNA, others .... X ──Q53

In general, do you go to the dentist for:

a regular check-up 1

an occasional check-up 2

Running prompt   or only when you are having trouble with your teeth? 3

Spontaneous only   never 4

52. People vary in how much trouble they have had with their teeth. How many of your teeth are currently filled:

none 1

1 - 4 filled teeth 2

Running prompt   5 or more filled teeth 3

or do you have no natural teeth? 4

53. Finally, is there anything further you would like to add about ...... (CHILD'S) teeth, that I have not covered already?

No 1

Yes (specify, do not probe) 2

Enter
Finish Time
(24 hr clock)

Hrs	Mins

THANK INFORMANT FOR THEIR CO-OPERATION

Dental show cards

CARD A

1. Every night
2. 4 - 6 nights a week
3. 1 - 3 nights a week
4. Less often than once a week
5. Never

CARD B

a. Milk drinks
b. Fruit juices and squashes
c. Blackcurrant drinks
d. Fizzy drinks
e. Tea / coffee
f. Water
g. Herbal drinks / tea
h. Other (please specify)

CARD C

1. Less often than once a week
2. At least once a week but not every day
3. Once a day
4. More than once a day

Dietary interview schedule

IN CONFIDENCE

1340/W4 : YOUNG CHILDREN'S DIETARY SURVEY

(C)

Serial no. label

Interviewer name ....

Authorisation no. ....

	Day	Month	Year
Date of Interview			9 3

	Hours	Mins
Enter start time - 24 hr clock		

- - - - - - - - - - - - - - - -

INTERVIEWER CODE

(a) Who was interviewed as informant

Code one only

Child's mother (female parent- figure) 1

Child's father (male parent- figure) 2

Child's 'mother' and 'father' jointly 3

Enter per. no of informant(s) →

Details of selected child

First name	Sex M F	Age	Date of birth Day Mth Year	Fam. unit
	1 2			①

List other household members in relationship to selected child

Person no. Ring →	Relationship to selected CHILD	OFF USE B	HOH Ring →	Sex M F	Age	Marital Status M C S W/D/S
⓪1			①	1 2		1 2 3 4
02				1 2		1 2 3 4
03				1 2		1 2 3 4
04				1 2		1 2 3 4
05				1 2		1 2 3 4
06				1 2		1 2 3 4
07				1 2		1 2 3 4
08				1 2		1 2 3 4
09				1 2		1 2 3 4
10				1 2		1 2 3 4

Fam. unit

1. **Applies if child's mother is married or cohabiting with no husband/partner in household**

Is (your husband) absent because he usually works away from home, or for some other reason?

DNA, others X

Usually works away 1 Q2
Inc. Armed Forces & Merchant Navy

Some other reason (specify) 2 Q2

2

PRESENT ACCOMMODATION

Ring codes at Q2 and Q3

2. Type of accommodation occupied by **this household**:

Code one from observation, if in doubt ask informant

whole house, bungalow	1	→ Q4
purpose-built flat or maisonette in block	2	→ Q3
part of the house/converted flat or maisonette/rooms in house	3	
dwelling with business premises	4	→ Q4
caravan/houseboat	5	
Other (specify)	6	

3. To households coded 2 - 4

What is the floor level of the main living part of the accommodation?

Basement/semi-basement	1
Ground floor/street level	2
1st floor	3
2nd floor	4
3th floor	5
4th to 9th floor	6
10th floor or higher	7

4. Ask or record

Is there a garden or other area attached to your accommodation where...........(CHILD) could play outside?

Yes	1
No	2

3

5. Do you have a kitchen, that is a separate room in which you cook?

Yes	1	(a)
No	2	(b)

(a) Do you share the kitchen with any other household?

Yes	1	Q6
No	2	

(b) Are you able to cook a hot meal in this accommodation?

Yes, hot meal	1
No	2
Spontaneous: Hot drink only	3

6. Does your household have any of the following items in your (part of the) accommodation?

INCLUDE: Items stored and under repair

	Yes	No
Refrigerator?	1	2
Deep freezer or fridge freezer?	1	2
Microwave oven?	1	2

7. Is there a car or van **normally** available for use by you or any members of your household?

Yes	1	(a)
No	2	Q8

INCLUDE: Any provided by employers if normally available for private use by informant or members of the household. EXCLUDE: Vehicles used solely for the carriage of goods.

(a) Is there one or more than one?

1	1	
2	2	Q8
3 or more	3	

4

Dietary interview schedule -continued

EATING HABITS: Introduce

8. Do you find .... (CHILD) particularly easy, about average or particularly difficult to feed for a child of his/her age?

* Easy	1	(a)
Average	2	**Q9**
Difficult	3	(a)

If easy or difficult
(a) In what way is (he/she) (easy/difficult) to feed?

9. How would you describe the variety of foods that .... (CHILD) generally eats? Does he/she

* **Running prompt** eat most things	1
eat a reasonable variety of things......	2
or is he/she a fussy or faddy eater?..	3

10. Does .... (CHILD) have

* **Running prompt** a good appetite	1
an average appetite...................	2
or a poor appetite	3
for a child of his/her age?	

11. Do you ever eat any food from .... (CHILD'S) plate to encourage him/her to eat it?

Yes.................	1	(a)
No	2	**Q12**

(a) How often do you do this? Is it

Running prompt most mealtimes..................	1
some mealtimes	2
or very occasionally?	3

12. And does .... (CHILD) ever eat any food from your (or anyone else's) plate?

Yes.................	1	(a)
No	2	**Q13**

(a) How often does this happen? Is it

Running prompt most mealtimes..................	1
some mealtimes	2
or very occasionally?.................	3

13. Are there any foods that .... (CHILD) does not eat because he/she does not like them?

Yes.................	1	**Specify**
No	2	**Q14**

IF YES SPECIFY WHICH FOODS

Dietary interview schedule -continued

14. Do you avoid giving ....(CHILD) particular foods or drinks because he/she is allergic to them?

Yes...........1   (a) - (c)

No...........2   Q15

If yes

(a) Which foods do you avoid?

Specify

(b) What form does the allergy take?   **(b)**

Specify

(c) Has ....(CHILD'S) allergy been diagnosed by a doctor?   **(c)**

Yes...........1

No...........2

15. (Apart from these) Are there any (other) foods you do not give ....(CHILD) for health, religious or any other reasons?

Yes...........1   (a)

No...........2   Q16

(a) **If yes specify which foods and give reasons**

FOOD   REASON

7

16. I'd like to ask you about what your child usually has to eat at different times of the day, but first I'd like to find out what times he/she gets up, has breakfast, has lunch and so on.

At what time approximately does ....(CHILD) usually ....(EVENT)

Prompt each event for time on weekdays, on Saturdays and on Sundays. Record approx. times in the grid.

Event	Weekdays	Saturdays	Sundays
gets up on ....at:			
has breakfast on ....at:			
has lunch on ....at:			
has tea on ....at:			
goes to bed on ....at:			

17. I'd now like to know, in general terms, what ....(CHILD) usually has to eat and drink at these different times. For example, at breakfast, does he/she have cereal, or toast, or a cooked breakfast? Some children don't eat breakfast, so if ....(CHILD) does not have anything at a particular time, please tell me.

What does he/she usually have to eat and drink, if anything ....

Prompt each event for what eaten on weekdays, on Saturdays and on Sundays. Record brief description in grid.

Event	Weekdays	Saturdays	Sundays
in bed or before breakfast on	Nil..........x	Nil..........x	Nil..........x

8

Dietary interview schedule -*continued*

Event	Weekdays	Saturdays	Sundays
for breakfast on	Nil x	Nil x	Nil x
during the morning on	Nil x	Nil x	Nil x
for lunch on	Nil x	Nil x	Nil x
during the afternoon on	Nil x	Nil x	Nil x
for tea on	Nil x	Nil x	Nil x
between tea and bed-time on	Nil x	Nil x	Nil x
in bed or during the night on	Nil x	Nil x	Nil x

DRINKING

18. Does . . . . . (CHILD) usually drink from

a feeder beaker/beaker with spout	1	⌉
a plastic cup or beaker	2	⎬ Q19
an ordinary cup, mug or glass	3	⌋
a bottle	4	— Q20
or from something else? (specify)	5	— Q19

Running prompt

19. (May I check) Does . . . . . (CHILD) have a bottle at all these days, even just to go to bed with?

Include ALL drinks given in a bottle

Yes, has a bottle	1	— Q20
No, never has a bottle	2	— Q21

20. On average, how many bottles does . . . . . (CHILD) have a day?

Include ALL drinks given in a bottle

Prompt as necessary

Fewer than 1 a day	00
1 a day	01
2 a day	02
3 a day	03
4 a day	04
More than 4 a day (specify)	—

Dietary interview schedule -continued

21. Does .....(CHILD) drink tea?

Yes.........	1	**(a)**
No..........	2	**Q22**

(a) Does .....(CHILD) usually take sugar in tea, is it sweetened with an artificial sweetener, or does .....(CHILD) drink tea without sugar or sweetener?

Sugar in tea.....	1
Artificial sweetener in tea.....	2
Drinks tea unsweetened.....	3

22. (May I check) does your child drink herbal teas <u>or</u> herbal infant drinks?

Yes, drinks herbal teas <u>or</u> herbal infant drinks.....	1	**(a)(b)**
No, drinks neither.....	2	**Q23**

(a) <u>On average</u>, how often does .....(CHILD) drink herbal tea or have a herbal infant drink?

[Show card A]

More than once a day.....	1
Once a day.....	2
Most days.....	3
At least once a week.....	4
At least once a month.....	5
Less than once a month.....	6

(b) What brands of herbal tea or herbal infant drink are you giving your child at the moment?

Record full brand name **and flavour** of all herbal teas/herbal infant drinks being given

1. ....
2. ....
3. ....

Write in number of brands ⟶ [ ]

11

---

23. Does .....(CHILD) drink coffee?

Yes.........	1	**(a)**
No..........	2	**Q24**

(a) Does .....(CHILD) usually take sugar in coffee, is it sweetened with an artificial sweetener, or does .....(CHILD) drink coffee without sugar or sweetener?

Sugar in coffee.....	1
Artificial sweetener in coffee.....	2
Drinks coffee unsweetened.....	3

24. (Apart from in tea and coffee) do you use artificial sweeteners to sweeten any of .....(CHILD'S) food, **either at the table or in cooking?**

Yes, uses artificial sweeteners.....	1	**(a)**
No, does not use artificial sweeteners.....	2	**Q25**

(a) Do you use an artificial sweetener, **either at the table or in cooking,** to sweeten .....(ITEM) for .....(CHILD)?

Prompt each food item and code in grid

	Yes used	Not used	Not eaten
Stewed or cooked fruit.....	1	2	9
Fresh fruit.....	1	2	9
Breakfast cereals.....	1	2	9
Cakes, biscuits or pastry that are homemade.....	1	2	9
Drinks, **other than** tea or coffee.....	1	2	9
Any other food or drink (specify).....	1	2	9
....	1	2	9

12

Dietary interview schedule -continued

25. Applies if any artificial sweetener used
for child:

    Code 1 AT Q24 (any food)
    Code 2 AT Q23(a) (in coffee)
    Code 2 AT Q21(a) (in tea)

DNA, no artificial sweeteners used ....X | ------- | Q26

What brands of artificial sweetener are you using to sweeten
.... (CHILD'S) food and drinks at the moment?

**Record full name and type - tablet, liquid, granulated,
of all artificial sweeteners being used for child**

1. ....

2. ....

3. .... | :.......... | **Write in number of brands** ⟶ |

26. Do you usually add salt to .... (CHILD'S) food **during cooking?**

Yes, includes sea salt...............	1
Yes, uses 'Lo Salt'/salt alternative (not sea salt)	2
No, does not use salt in cooking	3
Other (specify)	4
....	

27. **At the table**, do you add salt to .... (CHILD'S) food:

Running prompt usually	1
occasionally	2
rarely	3
or never?	4

If **uses** 'Lo salt' or salt alternative (not sea salt) at table
ring code 1 - 3 **and** ring code ⟶ | 1 |

---

28. I would now like to ask you about some foods your child may eat.
Can you tell me about how often, on average,.... (CHILD) eats these foods.
Please choose your answer from this card.

Hand informant Card A | Prompt each food listed below and code in grid. For 'seasonal foods' eg ice cream, prompt if necessary ".......... *at this time of year*".

	More than once a day	Once a day	Most days	At least once a week	At least once a month	Less than once a month	Never
Breakfast cereals	1	2	3	4	5	6	7
Cakes	1	2	3	4	5	6	7
Biscuits - any	1	2	3	4	5	6	7
Chocolate - confectionery	1	2	3	4	5	6	7
Other sweets	1	2	3	4	5	6	7
Ice cream or ice lollies	1	2	3	4	5	6	7
Yogurt (flavoured or plain but not fromage frais)	1	2	3	4	5	6	7
Cheese or cheese spread (not fromage frais)	1	2	3	4	5	6	7
Milk (dairy)	1	2	3	4	5	6	7
Eggs (include in home cooking)	1	2	3	4	5	6	7
Blackcurrant only drinks	1	2	3	4	5	6	7
Fruit juice (not squash)	1	2	3	4	5	6	7
Fizzy drinks (not mineral water)	1	2	3	4	5	6	7
Fish or shellfish, including fish fingers	1	2	3	4	5	6	7
Sausages - British type	1	2	3	4	5	6	7
Liver - not products	1	2	3	4	5	6	7
Beef, eg as a roast, steak or mince, in stews etc	1	2	3	4	5	6	7
Lamb, eg as a roast or chops, in stews etc	1	2	3	4	5	6	7
Pork, eg as a roast or chops, in stews etc	1	2	3	4	5	6	7
Chicken and poultry, eg as a roast, in casseroles	1	2	3	4	5	6	7

Dietary interview schedule -continued

28. (cont).

	More than once a day	Once a day	Most days	At least once a week	At least once a month	Less than once a month	Never
Baked beans - canned	1	2	3	4	5	6	7
Peas, in any form	1	2	3	4	5	6	7
Leafy green vegetables eg. spring greens, sprouts, broccoli	1	2	3	4	5	6	7
Chips	1	2	3	4	5	6	7
Other potatoes	1	2	3	4	5	6	7
Fresh fruit (any)	1	2	3	4	5	6	7

29. And how often, on average, does . . . . (CHILD) eat each of these foods?

Show Card A Prompt each food listed and code in grid.
For 'seasonal foods' prompt if necessary "at this time of year".

	More than once a day	Once a day	Most days	At least once a week	At least once a month	Less than once a month	Never	Skin eaten? (a) Yes	No
Raw carrots	1	2	3	4	5	6	7	1	2
Cooked carrots	1	2	3	4	5	6	7	1	2
Other root vegetables, apart from carrots and potatoes e.g. parsnips, turnips, swedes	1	2	3	4	5	6	7	1	2
Button or baby mushrooms	1	2	3	4	5	6	7	1	2
Other mushrooms	1	2	3	4	5	6	7	1	2
Apples (fresh)	1	2	3	4	5	6	7	1	2
Pears (fresh)	1	2	3	4	5	6	7	1	2
Soft fruit (e.g. peaches, nectarines, grapes)	1	2	3	4	5	6	7	1	2
Citrus fruits (e.g. orange, tangerines,satsumas)	1	2	3	4	5	6	7	1	2
Fresh tomatoes	1	2	3	4	5	6	7	1	2
Cucumber	1	2	3	4	5	6	7	1	2

If child eats any of above ask for each food eaten

(a) Can you tell me whether . . . . . (CHILD) usually eats the skin on . . . . . (ITEM) ——

15

30. Applies if child ever eats potatoes or chips (see Q28)

DNA, never eats potatoes or chips . . . . [1] — Q31

Does your child eat the skin on . . . . . (TYPE OF POTATO) always, sometimes or never?

Prompt each type of potato listed below and code in grid.

	Eaten with skin left on			
	Always	Sometimes	Never	Never eaten
Baked/jacket potatoes (cooked without fat)	1	2	3	4
Boiled new potatoes	1	2	3	4
Boiled old potatoes	1	2	3	4
Roast potatoes (in fat)	1	2	3	4
Fried potatoes or chips	1	2	3	4

16

31. A lot of shops and supermarkets are selling foods which are labelled as 'organic' or 'organically grown', what do you understand by the term 'organic' or organically grown?

[*]

32. Do you buy any 'organic' foods for your child?

Yes .... 1 (a)

No 2 Q33

(a) Do you buy organic . . . . . (ITEM) for your child always, sometimes or never?

Prompt each food listed below and code in grid.

Buys for child	Always	Sometimes	Never
Organic fruit	1	2	3
Organic vegetables incl dried beans or lentils	1	2	3
Organic cereal products, rice, muesli, pasta etc	1	2	3
Meat	1	2	3
Anything else (specify)	1	2	3
	1	2	3

17

33. Do you grow any of your own fruit and vegetables, either in your garden or on an allotment?

Include : salad vegetables

Exclude : herbs

Yes .... 1 (a)(b)

No 2 Q34

(a) Do you grow them without using pesticides?

Yes, all 1

Yes, some 2

No, none 3

(b) Do you grow them without using artificial fertilizers?

Yes, all 1

Yes, some 2

No, none 3

34. Does . . . . (CHILD) ever put soil into his/her mouth or eat soil these days?

Yes 1

No 2

35. Thinking about any food you have in the house today, which of the following items do you have here today?

Prompt each type of food listed below and code in grid

	Has in house	Does not have in house
A breakfast cereal	1	2
Bread, or bread rolls	1	2
Milk, or liquid or powdered baby milk	1	2
A tin of baked beans or spaghetti	1	2
Eggs	1	2
Biscuits, of any kind	1	2
Potatoes	1	2
Chocolate, of any kind	1	2
Other sweets	1	2

18

Dietary interview schedule -continued

36. Thinking now about different foods that come in cans.

How long, on average, would you keep ....(ITEM) in an opened can before eating/drinking it/them?

Show Card B

Prompt each type of food and code in grid below

	Code from Card B					Spontaneous only	
	More than a week	4 or 5 days	2 or 3 days	1 day	Use on same day	Never stored in open can	Not eaten/ drunk
Canned soft drinks eg cola, lemonade	1	2	3	4	5	6	7
Canned fruit juice	1	2	3	4	5	6	7
Baked beans	1	2	3	4	5	6	7
Spaghetti	1	2	3	4	5	6	7
Canned soup	1	2	3	4	5	6	7
Corned beef	1	2	3	4	5	6	7
Canned fish, eg, sardines, tuna	1	2	3	4	5	6	7

19

---

37. At present are you giving........(CHILD) fluoride tablets or drops?

Yes 1
No 2

38. And at present (apart from fluoride tablets/drops) are you giving ....(CHILD) any extra vitamins or minerals, as tablets, pills, powders, syrups or drops?

Yes 1
No 2

39. Applies if taking fluoride tablets/drops and/or supplements.

DNA X
(Qns 37 &38 coded No)

Q40

For each type taken record full description from bottle, including brand name and product licence number; record dose given to the child; how often taken, and form.

| WRITE IN BLOCK CAPITALS | INCLUDE FLUORIDE |

SUPPLEMENT 1	SUPPLEMENT 2
Full name , incl brand:	Full name , incl brand:
Office use only	*Office use only*
Dose: no. of tablets, drops, 5ml spoons:	Dose: no. of tablets, drops, 5ml spoons:
Office use only	*Office use only*
Frequency: no. of times and period eg 3 x day	Frequency: no. of times and period eg 3 x day
Office use only	*Office use only*
Form: ring code Drops .... 1 Pills/tablets ..... 2 Liquid/syrup ...... 3 Powder 4	Form: ring code Drops .... 1 Pills/tablets ..... 2 Liquid/syrup ...... 3 Powder 4
Product licence number (if any)	Product licence number (if any)
PL.:	PL.:

20

Dietary interview schedule -continued

Q39. (cont.)

SUPPLEMENT 3

Full name , incl brand: *Office use only*

Dose: no. of tablets, drops, 5ml spoons: *Office use only*

Frequency: no. of times and period
eg 3 x day   *Office use only*

Form: ring code

Drops	1
Pills/tablets	2
Liquid/syrup	3
Powder	4

Product licence number (if any)

PL:

SUPPLEMENT 4

Full name , incl brand: *Office use only*

Dose: no. of tablets, drops, 5ml spoons: *Office use only*

Frequency: no. of times and period
eg 3 x day   *Office use only*

Form: ring code

Drops	1
Pills/tablets	2
Liquid/syrup	3
Powder	4

Product licence number (if any)

PL:

SUPPLEMENT 5

Full name , incl brand: *Office use only*

Dose: no. of tablets, drops, 5ml spoons: *Office use only*

Frequency: no. of times and period
eg 3 x day   *Office use only*

Form: ring code

Drops	1
Pills/tablets	2
Liquid/syrup	3
Powder	4

Product licence number (if any)

PL:

SUPPLEMENT 6

Full name , incl brand: *Office use only*

Dose: no. of tablets, drops, 5ml spoons: *Office use only*

Frequency: no. of times and period
eg 3 x day   *Office use only*

Form: ring code

Drops	1
Pills/tablets	2
Liquid/syrup	3
Powder	4

Product licence number (if any)

PL:

CHILD'S MEDICAL HISTORY

40. Code or ask:

Is informant child's natural mother?

Yes 1   Q41
No 2   (a)

(a) Code or ask:

Is child's natural mother in the household?

Yes 1   Q41
No 2

41. Thinking back to when . . . . . (CHILD) was born, was he/she born prematurely or early?

Don't know 9   Q42
Yes/ yes - qualified answer 1   (a)
No 2   Q42

(a) How many weeks premature (early) was he/she?

[*] Less than 1 week 00
Other: specify no. of weeks .... [......]

42. How much did (s)he weigh at birth?

Pounds   ounces

OR

Grams

Don't know/can't remember 1   see Q43

Dietary interview schedule -continued

43. Applies if informant is child's natural mother, (Qn 40 coded 1)

DNA, informant is **not** child's natural mother ....X — Q44

Can I just check, how many children have **you** had, I mean all those who are living now (no matter what age) plus any who have died since birth including ..... (CHILD)?

> Exclude stillborn, step, adopted and foster children

Record number ↑ ....:......

DNA, only one child ......X — Q44

Record birth order number → ......:...... Q44

(a) **If more than one ask**
Was ..... (CHILD) your first child, your second (or which)?

44. Has ..... (CHILD) ever had an accident which resulted in a hospital admission?

Yes......1
No......2

45. Has ..... (CHILD) ever had an operation?

Yes......1
No......2

46. Has ..... (CHILD) ever stayed in hospital as an inpatient, overnight or longer?

Yes......1
No......2

> Exclude period after birth unless baby stayed in hospital after mother had left

47. We would like to know about bowel movements of young children (as this is linked to their diets and health). How many times did ..... (CHILD) open his/her bowels yesterday?

Don't know ....09 — Q48
None ....00 — Q49
Write in number of times → ......:...... — Q48

23

---

48. Yesterday was his/her poo/stool normal for him/her or abnormal?

normal ....1 — Q49
abnormal ....2] (a)
some normal, some abnormal ....3]

	Yes	No
(a) In what way was it abnormal? Was it		
a different colour to normal?	1	2
runnier than normal?	1	2
Individual prompt harder than normal?	1	2
smellier than normal?	1	2
abnormal in any other way? (specify)	1	2

49. Applies if informant is child's **natural mother**

DNA, informant is not child's natural mother.............X — Q50

I'd like to ask you about how you fed ..... (CHILD) when he/she was a baby. Did you ever put .....(CHILD) to the breast?

Yes (even only once) ....1 — (a)(b)
No ....2 — Q51

(a) For how long did you continue breast feeding ..... (CHILD)?

Please <u>include</u> the time when you were giving breast feeds <u>and</u> other feeds.

☐☐ days
or ☐☐ weeks
or ☐☐ months

> Record days
> or weeks
> or months

(b) Did you **ever** give ..... (CHILD) baby or infant formula milk, or follow-on milk, like Progress or Junior Milk?

Yes ....1 — Q51
No, never ....2 — Q53

24

Dietary interview schedule - *continued*

50. Can I check, when .....(CHILD) was a baby did (s)he ever have baby or infant formula milk, or follow-on milk like Progress or Junior Milk (not liquid cow's milk)?

Yes	1	— Q51
No, never	2	
Don't know	3	— Q53

51. At present is .....(CHILD), having any baby or infant formula milk, or follow-on milk like Progress or Junior Milk, even just at bedtime?

[Exclude liquid cow's milk]

Yes	1	— Q53
No	2	— Q52

52. How old was .....(CHILD) when he/she stopped having any baby, infant, formula or follow-on milk even at bedtime?

[Exclude liquid cow's milk]

under 1 month	00
1 month - under 2 months	01
2 months - under 3 months	02
3 months - under 6 months	03
6 months - under 9 months	04
9 months - under 1 year	05
1 year - under 1½ years	06
1½ years - under 2 years	07
2 years - under 2½ years	08
2½ years - under 3 years	09
3 years or older	10

Prompt as necessary

---

53. Nowadays, does .....(CHILD) have cow's milk as a drink?

Yes	1	(b)
No	2	(a)

(a) Has he/she ever had cow's milk as a drink?

Yes	1	(b)
No, never	2	Q54

(b) How old was .....(CHILD) when he/she started having cow's milk as a drink?

Code in grid at bottom of page

54. What kind of milk does ..... (CHILD) usually have as a drink these days?

Prompt as necessary

Whole milk	01	Q55
Semi-skimmed milk	02	
Skimmed milk	03	(a)
Powdered baby milk	04	
Does not drink milk	05	Q55
Other (specify)	06	

(a) How old was .....(CHILD) when he/she first had .....(TYPE OF MILK) as a drink?

Prompt as necessary

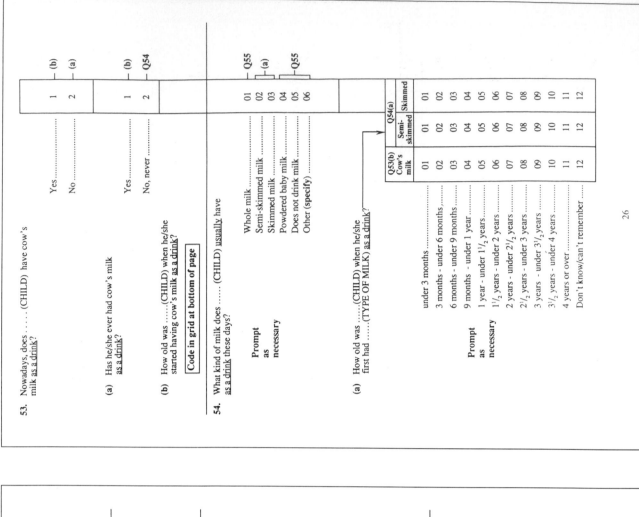

	Q53(b) Cow's milk	Q54(a) Semi-skimmed	Q54(a) Skimmed
under 3 months	01	01	01
3 months - under 6 months	02	02	02
6 months - under 9 months	03	03	03
9 months - under 1 year	04	04	04
1 year - under 1½ years	05	05	05
1½ years - under 2 years	06	06	06
2 years - under 2½ years	07	07	07
2½ years - under 3 years	08	08	08
3 years - under 3½ years	09	09	09
3½ years - under 4 years	10	10	10
4 years or over	11	11	11
Don't know/can't remember	12	12	12

Dietary interview schedule -continued

55. Apart from as a drink, what kinds of milk do you give.....(CHILD) on cereal, in puddings etc?

Prompt as necessary

Code all that apply

Whole milk	01
Semi-skimmed milk	02
Skimmed milk	03
Powdered baby milk	04
Doesn't have any milk	05
Other (specify)	06

---

56. 'MOTHER'S' EMPLOYMENT

DNA, no mother/female parent-figure in household **1** → Q68

Did you do any paid work last week - that is in the seven days ending last Sunday - either as an employee or self-employed?

Yes ... 1 → Q57
No ... 2 → Q58

57. Were you working full or part time?

Full time = more than 30 hrs
Part time = 30 hrs or less

Full time ... 1
Part time ... 2 → Q62

58. Even though you were not working did you have a job that you were away from last week?

Yes, is on maternity leave ... 1 → Q62
Yes, has a job and is not on maternity leave ... 3 → Q62
No ... 2 → Q59

59. Last week were you:

Individual prompt

Code first that applies

waiting to take up a job that you had already obtained? ... 1 → Q60
looking for work? ... 2
intending to look for work but prevented by temporary sickness or injury? **(Check: 28 days or less)** ... 3
going to school or college full time? **(aged 16 - 49 only)** ... 4
permanently unable to work because of long-term sickness or disability? **(aged 16 - 59 only)** ... 5 → Q61
retired. **(only if stopped work after 50)** ... 6
looking after the home or family? ... 7
Or were you doing something else? **(specify)** ... 8

60. Apart from the job you are waiting to take up have you ever had a paid job or done any paid work?

Yes ... 1 → Q62
No ... 2

61. May I just check, have you ever had a paid job or done any paid work?

Yes ... 1 → Q62
No ... 2 → Q68

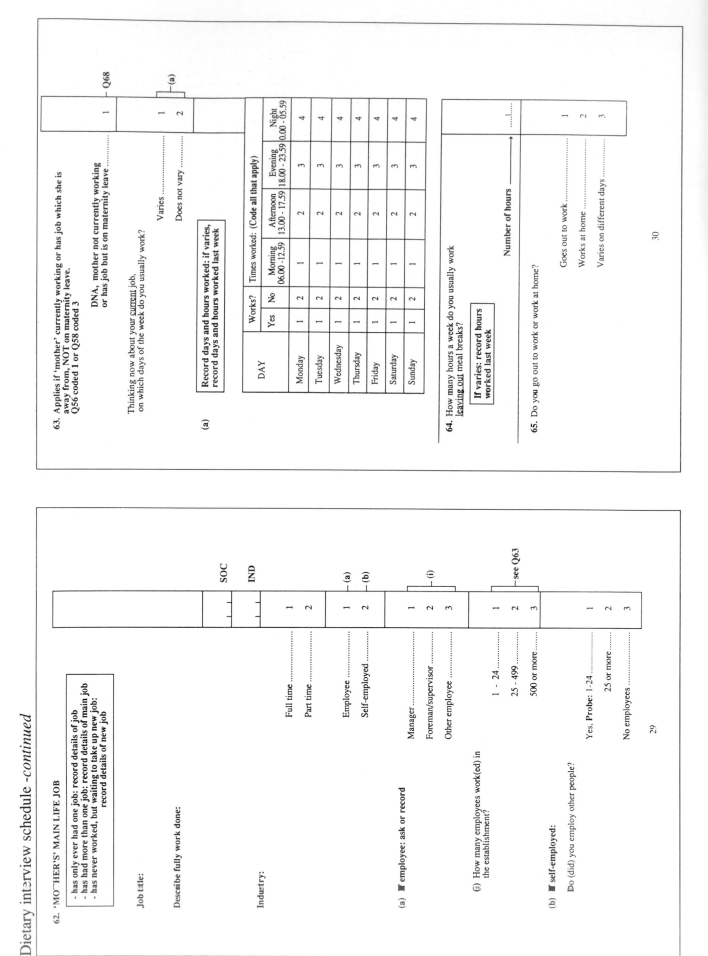

Dietary interview schedule -continued

62. 'MOTHER'S' MAIN LIFE JOB

- has only ever had one job: record details of job
- has had more than one job: record details of main job
- has never worked, but waiting to take up new job: record details of new job

Job title:

Describe fully work done:

SOC

IND

Industry:

Full time 1
Part time 2

Employee .... 1 (a)
Self-employed .... 2 (b)

(a) ▶ employee: ask or record

Manager .... 1 (i)
Foreman/supervisor 2
Other employee 3

(i) How many employees work(ed) in the establishment?

1 - 24 .... 1 see Q63
25 - 499 2
500 or more 3

(b) ▶ self-employed:

Do (did) you employ other people?

Yes, **Probe:** 1-24 1
25 or more 2
No employees 3

29

63. Applies if 'mother' currently working or has job which she is away from, NOT on maternity leave. Q56 coded 1 or Q58 coded 3

DNA, mother not currently working or has job but is on maternity leave ...... 1 — Q68

Thinking now about your current job, on which days of the week do you usually work?

Varies .... 1 —(a)
Does not vary 2

(a) **Record days and hours worked: if varies, record days and hours worked last week**

DAY	Works? Yes	Works? No	Times worked: (Code all that apply) Morning 06.00 -12.59	Afternoon 13.00 - 17.59	Evening 18.00 - 23.59	Night 0.00 - 05.59
Monday	1	2	1	2	3	4
Tuesday	1	2	1	2	3	4
Wednesday	1	2	1	2	3	4
Thursday	1	2	1	2	3	4
Friday	1	2	1	2	3	4
Saturday	1	2	1	2	3	4
Sunday	1	2	1	2	3	4

64. How many hours a week do you usually work leaving out meal breaks?

If varies: record hours worked last week

Number of hours ⟶ ....

65. Do you go out to work or work at home?

Goes out to work 1
Works at home 2
Varies on different days 3

30

Dietary interview schedule -continued

66. When you are working is .....(CHILD) usually looked after at home or away from home?

Looked after at home	1
Looked after away from home	2
Varies	3

> If sometimes at home, sometimes away, record place child spends most time while mother working

67. At present who looks after .....(CHILD) while you are working?

	Q67 All	Q67(a) Main
Child's 'mother', at home	01	01
Child's 'mother', takes child to work with her.	02	02
Child's 'father'	03	03
Child's grandparent	04	04
Code — Child's brother/sister	05	05
all — Other relative of child in household	06	06
that — Other relative of child outside household	07	07
apply — Friend/neighbour	08	08
Nanny	09	09
Paid childminder	10	10
Nurseryschool/class	11	11
School	12	12
Day Nursery or Creche	13	13
Play group	14	14
Other (specify)	15	15

(a) Applies if more than one person looks after child

Who mainly looks after .....(CHILD) while you are working?

Only one ...... X — — — Q68

Code in column above

31

---

68. TO ALL

Show Card C

At present, is ....(CHILD) going to any of these regularly each week?

Code those attended in grid below; INCLUDE any mentioned at Q67

None attended ...... 9 → see Q69

For each attended ask (a) - (d) and code in grid below

(a) On how many days a week does ....(CHILD) usually go to the ....(PLACE/PERSON)?

(b) Does he/she usually go there:
all day
mornings or afternoons only
or some other time?

Running prompt

(c) Does he/she usually have a meal while he/she is there?

(d) Does he/she usually have any drinks or snacks while he/she is there?

	Q68		Q68(a) No. of days/week child attends	Q68(b) Hours attended?			Q68(c) Meals?		Q68(d) Snacks?	
	Yes	No		all day	mornings or afternoons only	other	Yes	No	Yes	No
Play group/Play school	1	2		1	2	3	1	2	1	2
Mother and toddler group	1	2		1	2	3	1	2	1	2
Nursery school/class	1	2		1	2	3	1	2	1	2
Day nursery or creche	1	2		1	2	3	1	2	1	2
Primary/Infants school	1	2		1	2	3	1	2	1	2
Childminder	1	2		1	2	3	1	2	1	2
Other children's group or childcare (specify)	1	2		1	2	3	1	2	1	2
	1	2		1	2	3	1	2	1	2
	1	2		1	2	3	1	2	1	2

32

Dietary interview schedule -continued

69. 'FATHER'S' EMPLOYMENT (male parent-figure)
If no 'father' in household, ask about HOH

Enter per. no. from h'hold box ⟶

DNA, no 'father' and 'mother' is HOH .. 1 —— Q75 mother

Did (your husband/HOH) do any paid work last week,
that is in the seven days ending last Sunday, either
as an employee or self-employed?

Yes	1	Q74
No	2	Q70

70. Even though (he) was not working, did (he) have a
job that he was away from last week?

Yes	1	Q74
No	2	Q71

71. Last week was (he):

waiting to take up a job that (he) had already obtained?	1	Q72
Individual prompt looking for work?	2	
intending to look for work but prevented by temporary sickness or injury? **(Check: 28 days or less)**	3	
going to school or college full time? **(aged 16-49 only)**	4	Q73
Code first that applies permanently unable to work because of long-term sickness or disability? **(men 16-64; women 16-59 only)**	5	
retired? **(for women, only if stopped work after age 50)**	6	
looking after the home or family?	7	
or was (he) doing something else? **(specify)**	8	

72. Apart from the job (he) is waiting to take up,
has (he) ever had a paid job or done any paid work?

Yes	1	Q74
No	2	Q75

73. May I just check, has (he) ever had a paid job,
or done any paid work?

Yes	1	Q74
No	2	Q75

33

---

74. 'FATHER'S'/HOH's CURRENT JOB

- has one job at present: record details of job
- has more than one job at present: record details of **main** job
- is not currently working: record details of last job
- is waiting to take up job: record details of 'new job'

Job title:

Describe fully work done:

Industry:

	SOC	
		IND

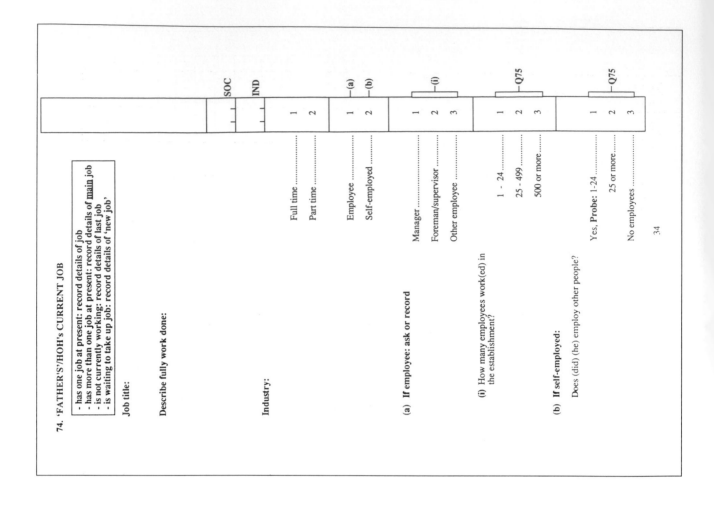

Full time	1	
Part time	2	
Employee	1	(a)
Self-employed	2	(b)
Manager	1	(i)
Foreman/supervisor	2	
Other employee	3	

(a) If employee: ask or record

(i) How many employees work(ed) in
the establishment?

1 - 24	1	Q75
25 - 499	2	
500 or more	3	

(b) If self-employed:

Does (did) (he) employ other people?

Yes, **Probe:** 1-24	1	Q75
25 or more	2	
No employees	3	

34

Dietary interview schedule -*continued*

75. 'PARENTS' EDUCATION

Ask Qns 75 and 76 about 'mother' and 'father' if present in household

	Mother figure	Father figure
Enter per no.		
DNA, no 'mother'	X	
DNA, no 'father'		X — Q76

How old were you (was your husband) when you (he) finished your (his) continuous full-time education?

	Mother figure	Father figure
Not yet finished	1	1
14 or under	2	2
15	3	3
16	4	4
17	5	5
18	6	6
19 or over	7	7
No formal education	8	8

35

---

76. Please look at this card and tell me whether you (your husband) have (has) any of the qualifications listed. Start at the top of the list and tell me the first one you come to that you have/he has passed

Show Card D

	Mother figure	Father figure
Degree (or degree level qualification)	1	1
Teaching qualification		
HNC/HND, BEC/TEC Higher, BTEC Higher		
City and Guilds Full Technological Certificate		
Nursing qualifications (SRN, SCM, RGN, RM RHV, Midwife)	2	2
'A' levels/SCE higher		
ONC/OND/BEC/TEC **not** higher	3	3
City and Guilds Advanced/Final		
Code first that applies		
'O' level passes (Grades A-C if after 1975)		
GCSE (Grades A-C)		
CSE (Grade 1)		
SCE Ordinary (Bands A-C)		
Standard Grade (Levels 1-3)	4	4
SLC Lower		
SUPE Lower or Ordinary		
School Certificate or Matric		
City and Guilds Craft/Ordinary level		
CSE Grades 2-5		
GCE 'O' level (Grades D & E if after 1975)		
GCSE (Grades D, E, F, G)		
SCE Ordinary (Bands D & E)	5	5
Standard Grade (Level 4, 5)		
Clerical or commercial qualifications		
Apprenticeship		
CSE ungraded	6	6
Other qualifications (specify)	7	7
No qualifications	8	8

36

Dietary interview schedule -continued

77. Do you (does your husband) smoke cigarettes at all?

	Mother figure	Father figure
Yes	1	1
No	2	2

Applies if mother/father smoke

(a) About how many cigarettes a day do you (does he) usually smoke?

	Mother figure	Father figure
Less than 1	00	00
No. smoked a day →		
Don't know	99	99

78. 'MOTHER'S' PLACE OF BIRTH - female parent figure

	Mother figure	Father figure
DNA, no 'mother'	X	Q80

In which country were you born?

England	1
Scotland	2
Wales	3
N Ireland	4
Outside UK	5

79. To which of the groups listed as this card do you consider you belong?

Show Card E

White	1	
Black - Caribbean	2	Q80
Black - African	3	
Black - Other	4	(a)
Indian	5	
Pakistani	6	Q80
Bangladeshi	7	
Chinese	8	
None of these (include mixed race)	9	(a)

(a) How would you describe the racial or ethnic group to which you belong?

80. Does your household own or rent this house or flat?

Owns - with mortgage/loan	01
- outright	02
Rents - local authority/new town	03
- housing association	04
- privately unfurnished	05
- privately furnished	06
- from employer	07
- other with payment	08
Rent free	09

Prompt as necessary

81. Can I just check are you (or your husband) currently receiving Family Credit?

| Yes | 1 |
| No | 2 |

82. And have you (or your husband) drawn Income Support at any time in the last 14 days?

| Yes | 1 |
| No | 2 |

83. Could you please look at this card and tell me which group represents the gross income of the whole household?

Please include income from all sources before any compulsory deductions such as income tax, national insurance and superannuation contributions.

Show Card F

Group number	
Don't know	88
Refused	99

Remind informant who is included in the household

84. Enter finish time for questionnaire

Hours	Mins.

24 hr. clock

Dietary interview schedule -*continued*

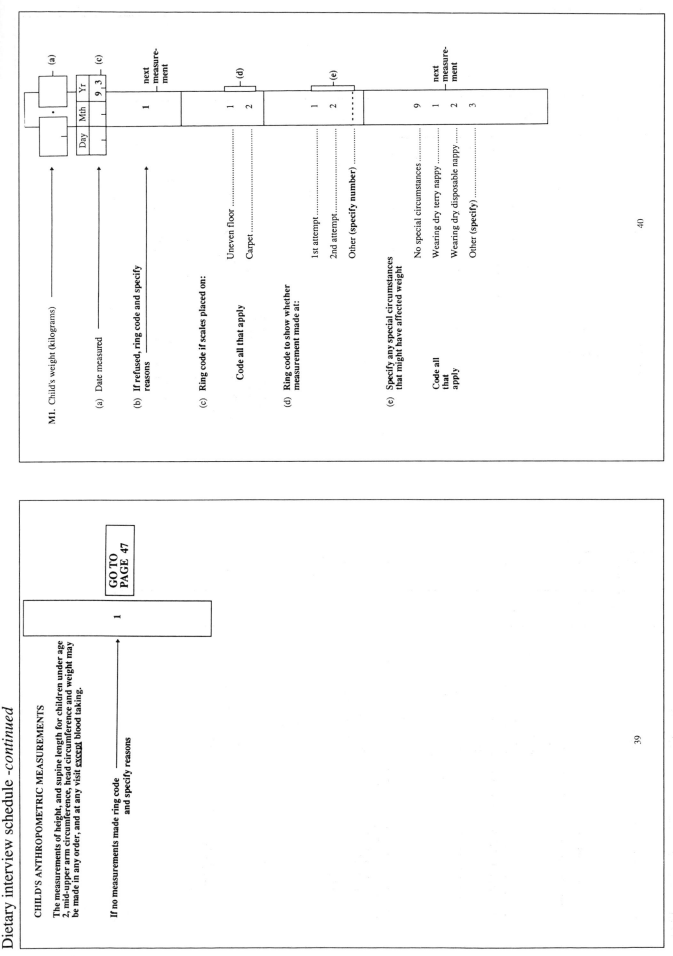

CHILD'S ANTHROPOMETRIC MEASUREMENTS

The measurements of height, and supine length for children under age 2, mid-upper arm circumference, head circumference and weight may be made in any order, and at any visit except blood taking.

If no measurements made ring code and specify reasons

1 → GO TO PAGE 47

39

M1. Child's weight (kilograms) — (a) [.]

(a) Date measured — (c) | Day | Mth | Yr | | | 9 | 3 |

(b) If refused, ring code and specify reasons — 1 next measurement

(c) Ring code if scales placed on:

    Code all that apply
    Uneven floor .... 1 (d)
    Carpet 2

(d) Ring code to show whether measurement made at:
    1st attempt .... 1 (e)
    2nd attempt 2
    Other (specify number) ....

(e) Specify any special circumstances that might have affected weight

    Code all that apply
    No special circumstances 9
    Wearing dry terry nappy .... 1 next measurement
    Wearing dry disposable nappy 2
    Other (specify) 3

40

Dietary interview schedule -*continued*

M2. Child's head circumference (cms) ⟶ (a)

Use standard tape

(a) Date measured ⟶

Day	Mth	Yr
		9 3

(c)

(b) If refused, ring code and specify reasons ⟶

    1 — next measure-ment

(c) Ring code to show whether measurement made at:

    1st attempt 1

    2nd attempt 2

    Other (specify number) .... (d)

(d) Specify any special circumstances that might have affected head circumference measurement

    No special circumstances .... 9 — next measure-ment

    Special circumstances (specify below) 1

41

M3. Child's mid upper arm circumference (mms) ⟶ (a)

Use TALC insertion tape

(a) Date measured ⟶

Day	Mth	Yr
		9 3

(c)

(b) If refused, ring code and specify reasons ⟶

    1 — next measure-ment

(c) Ring code to show whether measurement made at:

    1st attempt 1

    2nd attempt 2

    Other (specify number) .... (d)

(d) Specify any special circumstances that might have affected mid upper arm circumference measurement

    No special circumstances .... 9 — next measure-ment

    Special circumstances (specify below) 1

42

Dietary interview schedule -continued

M4. Child's standing height (m)

(a) Date measured

Day	Mth	Yr
		9 3

(b) If refused, ring code and specify reasons → 1   next measurement

(c) Ring code if standing height not measured because child under 0.750m → 1   next measurement

(d) Ring code to show whether measurement made at:

- 1st attempt....... 1
- 2nd attempt....... 2
- Other (specify number)....... (e)

(e) Ring code if height affected by

Code all that apply

- Height not affected....... 9
- Hairstyle....... 1
- Turban....... 2
- Posture - back not straight....... 3
- Posture - legs not straight....... 4
- Unable to stand still....... 5
- Other (specify)....... 6   next measurement

43

M5. Child's supine length (m)

Applies to children <u>under age 2 at time of measuring</u>

DNA, aged 2 or over....... 9   next measurement or M6

Supine length   .   (a)

> **Deduct 0.100 from Digi-Rod display if spacer block used**

(a) Date measured

Day	Mth	Yr
		9 3	(b)

(b) Ring code if spacer block used → 1 (d)

(c) If refused, ring code and specify reasons → 1 M6

(d) Ring code to show whether measurement made at:

- 1st attempt....... 1
- 2nd attempt....... 2
- Other (specify number)....... (e)

(e) Ring code if supine length affected by:

Code all that apply

- Supine length <u>not</u> affected....... 9
- Hairstyle....... 1
- Turban....... 2
- Posture - cannot lie flat....... 3
- Posture - cannot straighten legs....... 4
- Unable to lie still....... 5
- Other (specify)....... 6   next measurement or M6

44

Dietary interview schedule -*continued*

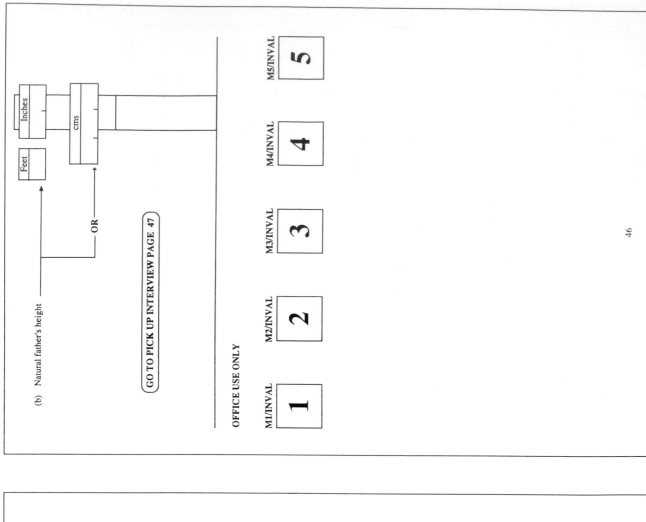

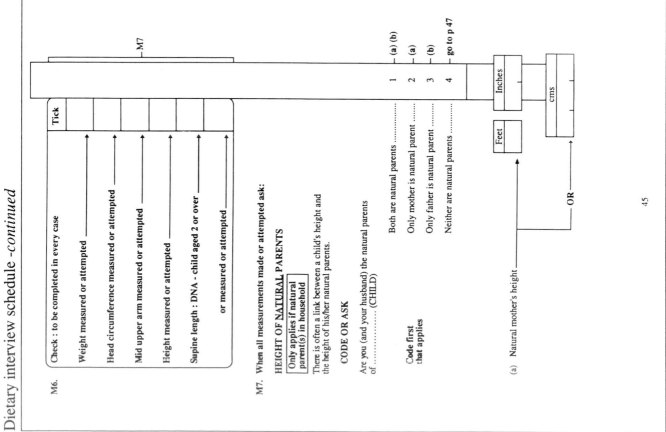

Dietary interview schedule -continued

FOLLOW-UP QUESTIONNAIRE TO BE ASKED AT PICK-UP CALL

F1. [Interviewer code]

Dietary record refused	1	—(a)
Partial dietary record	2	—F2
4 day dietary record	3	

(a) **Specify reasons dietary record refused/partial dietary record**

F2. Applies if partial or 4 day dietary record obtained

DNA, no dietary record ...... X ------- F23

[Interviewer code]

Bowel movements card fully/partially completed	1	—F3
No bowel movements card	2	—(a)

(a) **Specify reasons why no bowel movements card**

(GO TO F3)

47

Start time for follow-up questionnaire (use 24hr clock) →

Hours	Mins

F3. Record or ask

Who weighed and recorded the food and drink entered in the diary? Please include all those people who did any weighing and recording.

Code all that apply

	F3	(a)
Child's 'mother'	1	1
Child's 'father'	2	2
Child's brother(s) or sister(s)	3	3
Other relative of child	4	4
Nanny or childminder	5	5
Other (specify)	6	6
DNA, one person X		—F4

(a) **Applies if more than one person recording/weighing**

Who did most of the weighing and recording?

RING CODE IN COLUMN ABOVE

F4. Were there any foods that were impossible to weigh?

Yes	1	—(a)
No	2	—F5

(a) Which foods were these?

F5. Were there any situations, apart from when your child ate away from home, when it was not possible to weigh what your child was eating?

Yes	1	—(a)
No	2	—F6

(a) What situations were these?

48

Dietary interview schedule -continued

F6. Were there any occasions when you forgot to weigh and record any food or drink that your child had?

Yes .... 1 (a) (b) (c)
No 2 F7

(a) How often did this happen?

Several times a day 1
About once a day 2
Once or twice during the 4 days 3
Other (specify) 4
....

(b) What sorts of foods or drink did you forget to weigh?

(c) What did you do if you forgot to weigh something?

Prompt as necessary

Code all that apply

Missed it out completely 1
Put it in the diary with no weight 2
Weighed a similar item and entered this weight in the diary instead 3
Noted it down in the eating out diary 4
Other (specify) 5
....

F7. Do you consider your child to be a messy eater?

Yes .... 1 (a)
No 2 F9

(a) Did this cause you any problems with keeping the diary?

Yes .... 1 (i)
No 2 F8

(i) What sorts of problems did you have?

49

F8. If your child made a mess with their food did you manage to scrape it up and reweigh it as leftovers:

Running prompt

always 1
most of the time 2
only sometimes 3
or never? 4

F9. If your child ever left any of the food he/she was served, did you remember to weigh the leftovers and write the weight of them down in the diary:

Never any leftovers = code 1

Running prompt

always 1
most of the time 2
only sometimes 3
or never? 4

F10. If any food was wasted or eaten by someone else and therefore could not be reweighed as leftovers, did you remember to write this down in the diary:

Never wasted or eaten by somebody else = code 1

Running prompt

always 1
most of the time 2
only sometimes 3
or never? 4

50

Dietary interview schedule -continued

F11. During the (4) days that you were weighing and recording your child's food do you think you offered your child more, less or about the same amount of ....(ITEM) as usual?

Prompt each item listed below and code in the grid

	DNA, never eats item	Foods offered to your child		
		More	Less	Same
Biscuits	9	1	2	3
Sweets	9	1	2	3
Crisps	9	1	2	3
Drinks	9	1	2	3
Snacks	9	1	2	3

F12. On the whole, do you think that you offered your child:

Running prompt
bigger 1
smaller 2
or the same size portions as usual while you were keeping the diary? 3

F13. During the (4) days do you think your child ate out of the home including at friends or nursery:

Running prompt
more often 1
less often 2
or about the same as usual? 3

F14. While you were weighing and keeping the diary, did you give your child food that was easier to weigh than you would normally give him/her?

Yes, easier to weigh 1
No, same as usual 2

51

F15. Do you think you changed your child's normal diet in any other way during the time you were weighing his/her food?

Yes .... 1 — (a)
No .... 2 — F16

(a) In what way did you change your child's normal diet?

[*]

F16. Do you think you weighed and recorded the food more accurately at:

Running prompt
the beginning of the diary, ... 1
or towards the end of the diary 2
or was there no difference over the (4) days? 3

F17. Did you always weigh each item or did you sometimes copy down the weight from a previous occasion, for example, the weights of biscuits, drinks or any other item your child has regularly?

Weighed every item .... 1 — F18
Sometimes copied down weights......... 2 — (a)

(a) Which items were weights copied over from?

52

Dietary interview schedule -*continued*

F18. Ask or record

Did the eating out diary have to be left with someone else, for example a childminder or playgroup worker, for them to record food and drink eaten by your child?

Yes ...... 1 — (a)
No ...... 2 — F19

(a) Were there any problems in keeping the eating out diary when your child was with someone else?

Yes ...... 1 — (i)
No ...... 2 — F19

(i) What were these problems?
[symbol]

F19. Did you have any other problems with the weighing and recording of what your child had to eat and drink during the (4 day) period?

Yes ...... 1 — (a)
No ...... 2 — F20

(a) What were these problems?
[symbol]

53

F20. (During the past few days/while you were keeping the diary) has ....(CHILD) been unwell at all; has he/she:

Individual prompt	Yes	No
been teething?	1	2
had any diarrhoea?	1	2
been sick or vomited?	1	2
been unwell in any other way (specify)	1	2
......	1	2
......	1	2

DNA, not unwell during diary days .... 1 — F21

(a) Applies if any F20 coded 'yes'

On which day did he/she have (...... PROBLEM)

	Day 1	Day 2	Day 3	Day 4
DNA, not unwell this day	9	9	9	9
DNA, no diary this day	8	8	8	8
teething	1	1	1	1
diarrhoea	2	2	2	2
vomiting	3	3	3	3
other (specify)	4	4	4	4
......	5	5	5	5
......	6	6	6	6

(b) Ask for each day on which child was unwell

Did being unwell affect his/her eating habits on this day?

	Day 1	Day 2	Day 3	Day 4
Yes, eating affected......	1	1	1	1
No, eating not affected	2	2	2	2

RECORD COMMENTS AND PROBE AMBIGUTIES

54

Dietary interview schedule -*continued*

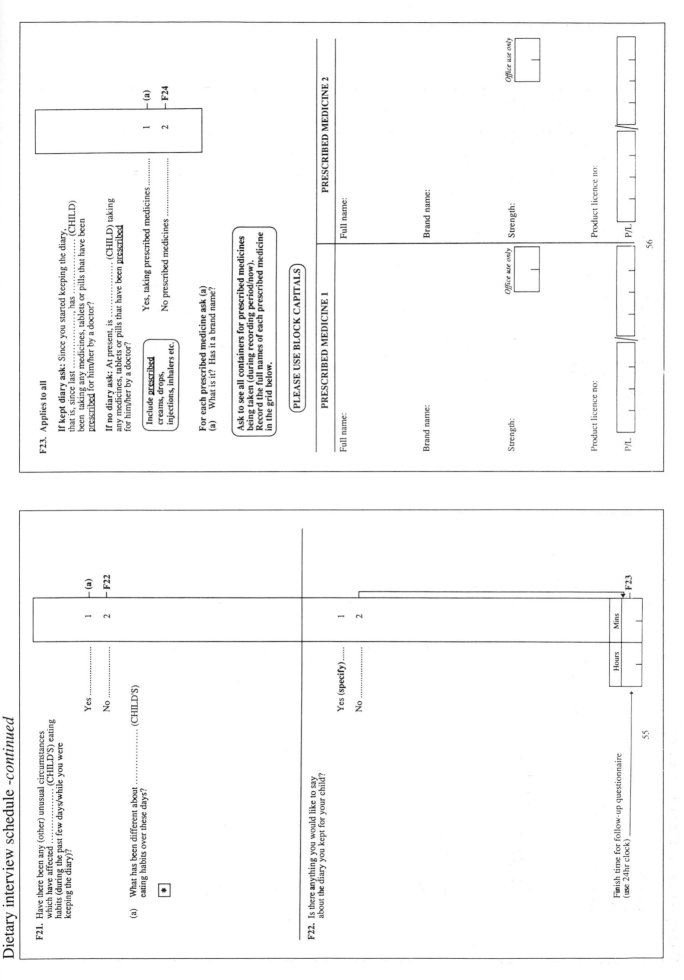

F21. Have there been any (other) unusual circumstances which have affected ....(CHILD'S) eating habits (during the past few days/while you were keeping the diary)?

Yes .... 1 **(a)**

No .... 2 ├── **F22**

(a) What has been different about ....(CHILD'S) eating habits over these days?

[*]

F22. Is there anything you would like to say about the diary you kept for your child?

Yes (**specify**) 1

No .... 2 ├── **F23**

Finish time for follow-up questionnaire (use 24hr clock)

Hours		Mins	

55

F23. Applies to all

If kept diary ask: Since you started keeping the diary, that is, since last ...., has .... (CHILD) been taking any medicines, tablets or pills that have been prescribed for him/her by a doctor?

If no diary ask: At present, is .... (CHILD) taking any medicines, tablets or pills that have been prescribed for him/her by a doctor?

┌─────────────────────────────┐
│ Include prescribed   │
│ creams, drops,   │
│ injections, inhalers etc.   │
└─────────────────────────────┘

Yes, taking prescribed medicines .... 1 **(a)**

No prescribed medicines .... 2 ├── **F24**

For each prescribed medicine ask (a)
(a) What is it? Has it a brand name?

┌──┐
│ Ask to see all containers for prescribed │
│ medicines being taken (during recording   │
│ period/now). Record the full names of   │
│ each prescribed medicine in the grid   │
│ below.   │
└──┘

(PLEASE USE BLOCK CAPITALS)

PRESCRIBED MEDICINE 1	PRESCRIBED MEDICINE 2
Full name:	Full name:
Brand name:	Brand name:
Strength: *Office use only*	Strength: *Office use only*
Product licence no:	Product licence no:
P/L	P/L

56

Dietary interview schedule -continued

PRESCRIBED MEDICINE 3

Full name:

Brand name:

Office use only

Strength:

Product licence no:

P/L

PRESCRIBED MEDICINE 4

Full name:

Brand name:

Office use only

Strength:

Product licence no:

P/L

PRESCRIBED MEDICINE 5

Full name:

Brand name:

Office use only

Strength:

Product licence no:

P/L

PRESCRIBED MEDICINE 6

Full name:

Brand name:

Office use only

Strength:

Product licence no:

P/L

PRESCRIBED MEDICINE 7

Full name:

Brand name:

Office use only

Strength:

Product licence no:

P/L

PRESCRIBED MEDICINE 8

Full name:

Brand name:

Office use only

Strength:

Product licence no:

P/L

57

F24. INTERVIEWER'S ASSESSMENT SHEET

To be completed in every case where diary kept.

DNA, no diary X

F25

Please record your own assessment of the quality of weighing and recording in the home record and eating out diary. Note any circumstances that you think might have affected eating habits or the quality of the diaries

58

Dietary interview schedule -*continued*

F25. INTERVIEWER'S PROGRESS CHECK		Tick if full or partial	Ring if DNA or refused
Collect: home record diary, with any wrappers	(E)	- - - -	X
eating out diary, with any wrappers	(F)	- - - -	X
bowel movements chart	(Q)	- - - -	X
Collect scales (and box) and bowl		- - - -	X
Complete incentive payment letter and form (**if 4 day diary**) (Y)		- - - -	X
Complete measurements of child		- - - -	X
Collect: measuring equipment:			
Scales		- - - -	X
TALC tape and pen		- - - -	X
Tape		- - - -	X
Digi-rod and block		- - - -	X
Record measurement of parents' height		- - - -	X

F26. To be completed after asking **dental recall** questions at final call

Copy code from Q1 on dental recall sheet

Yes, to interview and examination	1
Yes, to interview only	2
Yes, other/conditional	3
No	4
Dental recall qns not asked	5 — (a)

(a) **Specify** reasons why dental recall qns not asked

59

103

CARD A

N1340

1. More than once a day

2. Once a day

3. Most days

4. At least once a week, but not most days

5. At least once a month, but less often than

   once a week

6. Less than once a month

7. Never

CARD B

N1340

1. More than a week

2. No more than 4 or 5 days

3. No more than 2 or 3 days

4. No more than 1 day

5. Use on same day

CARD C

N1340

1. Playgroup or play school

2. Mother and toddler group

3. Nursery school or nursery class

4. Day nursery or creche

5. Primary or infants school

6. Childminder

7. Other children's group or childcare

CARD D

N1340

Degree (or degree level qualification)

Teaching qualification
HNC/HND, BEC/TEC Higher, BTEC Higher
City and Guilds Full Technological Certificate
Nursing qualifications (SRN, SCM, RGN, RM, RHV, Midwife)

'A' levels/SCE higher
ONC/OND/BEC/TEC not higher
City and Guilds Advanced/Final level

'O' level passes (Grade A-C if after 1975)
GCSE (grades A-C)
CSE Grade 1
SCE Ordinary (Bands A-C)
Standard Grade (Level 1-3)
SLC Lower
SUPE Lower or Ordinary
School Certificate or Matric
City and Guilds Craft/Ordinary level

CSE Grades 2-5
GCE 'O' level (Grades D&E if after 1975)
GCSE (Grades D,E,F,G)
SCE Ordinary (Bands D&E)
Standard Grade (Level 4,5)
Clerical or commercial qualifications
Apprenticeships

CSE ungraded

Other qualifications (specify)

No qualifications

CARD F

N1340

GROSS HOUSEHOLD INCOME

per week	Group	per year
less than £40	01	less than £2,000
£40 - less £80	02	£2,000 - less £4,000
£80 - less £120	03	£4,000 - less £6,000
£120 - less £160	04	£6,000 - less £8,000
£160 - less £200	05	£8,000 - less £10,000
£200 - less £240	06	£10,000- less £12,000
£240 - less £280	07	£12,000- less £14,000
£280 - less £350	08	£14,000- less £18,000
£350 - less £400	09	£18,000- less £20,000
£400 - less £500	10	£20,000- less £25,000
£500 - less £600	11	£25,000- less £30,000
£600 or more	12	£30,000 or more

CARD E

N1340

1. White
2. Black-Caribbean
3. Black-African
4. Black-Other
5. Indian
6. Pakistani
7. Bangladeshi
8. Chinese
9. None of these

Home record diary (E)

E

Serial no. label

Interviewer number ☐☐☐☐

CONFIDENTIAL
N1340/W4 NATIONAL DIET AND NUTRITION SURVEY;
CHILDREN AGED 1¹/₂ - 4¹/₂ YEARS

Sex
Boy   Girl
☐☐

Date of Birth
☐☐ ☐☐ ☐☐

HOME RECORD BOOK

Please record all food and drink
as shown inside. Thank you

The interviewer will call again on:

Day	Date	Time

Office of Population Censuses and Surveys
Social Survey Division
St Catherines House
10 Kingsway, London WC2B 6JP

107

Home Record Book

These instructions tell you how you to describe the food and drink items you weigh. You should also read the instructions at the front of the eating out diary.

Please read through all these notes carefully before starting the 4 days of weighing and recording. The interviewer will go over the main points with you, and can help with any difficulties you might have. The check list card is a quick reminder of how to use the scales and record food items.

DESCRIBING FOOD AND DRINK; as full a description of each food and drink, together with its brand name is needed.

Column A: Write down the time the food will be eaten, indicating whether the time was a.m. or p.m. Each plate entry should have a time written in this column. If you are preparing food for your child to take out of the home for lunch tomorrow, record the information on tomorrow's sheet.

Column B: Tick the first box if the food is being eaten at home; tick the second box if the food was eaten away from home.

Column C: Tick the first box if you are the child's mother or father recording the food and drink; tick the second box if you are someone else, eg the nanny, childminder, child's grandmother recording the food or drink.

Column D: Write down the brand or product name of the food. Please give as much information as possible. Describe each item ON A SEPARATE LINE. Fresh meat, fresh fish, fresh fruit and vegetables, doorstep milk, unwrapped bread and cakes and other fresh foods which are not pre-packed (cheese, cooked meats and pasta which are not pre-packed) do not need brand or product names. In these cases no information is required, so leave the space in this column blank. Do NOT write in the name of the shop where the item was bought. However, remember to record 'own brand' names in this column, eg Sainsbury's (baked beans).

Column E: Write down the description of the food. Please give as much information as possible - type of food, name, and how it was cooked. If the food was fried or roasted, please write down the type of fat or oil it was cooked in. If the food includes homemade pastry please write down the type of fat used to make the pastry. If the food was a bought dessert, for example, a yoghurt or fromage frais, write down what flavour it was and whether it was low fat, diet/ reduced sugar or not. If you need to, you may use more than one line, but please put EACH SEPARATE ITEM ON A SEPARATE LINE. If the item was a cooked dish made from several items, for example, Shepherd's pie, weigh the whole portion and describe it as Sheperd's pie in the diary. Do not try to weigh the potato and meat parts separately. Write down the recipe used to make the dish on the back of the previous page.

Column F: If the food item is fresh fruit or fresh vegetables please tick a box in this column against the item to show whether it was homegrown or not. By homegrown, we mean grown IN YOUR OWN GARDEN OR ALLOTMENT.

Column G: Write in the weight of the food or drink.

Column H: We need to know the weight of any leftovers, including any inedible parts, such as fruit stones or peel. You should weigh the plate with the leftovers on it and write the weight in column H next to the weight you wrote down for the empty plate. Make sure to put a tick next to each item of food left.

Column J: If something is spilt or eaten by someone other than the child and therefore not reweighed as leftovers, tick the box in column J. Write in the space along side the item about how much of the original item you think was lost; for example, "about ¹/₂ spilt". If it was a plateful of different foods that were spilt and you cannot estimate how much of each individual item was lost then bracket together all the items that were lost and estimate how much of the original plateful was lost.

For foods that already come in containers like yoghurt or trifles you can weigh the full container and then weigh the container again when your child has eaten the food. Or, if you prefer, you can tip out the food into a bowl which you have just weighed.

To weigh bread and butter or anything else you spread on bread, start by weighing the plate as usual. Press the button again to set the scale back to zero and weigh the bread. Press the button again to set the scale back to zero then remove the bread and quickly spread the butter. Put the bread back on the scales and it will show the weight of the butter or margarine you have just spread. Now set the scale back to zero and then remove the bread again to quickly spread the jam or marmalade. Put the bread back on the scale and it will show the weight of the jam you have put on. If the scales switch off before you have buttered your bread, or spread the filling, do not worry. Switch the scales on again and record the total weight of plate, bread, butter etc. However, please make a note against the entry to show what happened, for example, 'total weight of plate, one slice of toast, butter, marmalade'.

Children have a lot of drinks during the day. We need to know about ALL of them. If your child has a drink of squash, please weigh the concentrate and water separately and give a full description of the squash in column E. The 'Check List For Weighing' card has a step-by-step guide to weighing squash to help you.

Home record diary (E) - example page

A COMPLETED PAGE IN THE HOME RECORD BOOK SHOULD LOOK LIKE THIS

Day ...Friday...... day Date 0 3 0 7 9 2

		OFF. USE DAY OF WEEK	TICK A BOX TO SHOW WHETHER CHILD IS WELL OR UNWELL TODAY		Serial Number
			Well [√]1 Unwell [ ]2		

TICK A BOX TO SHOW WHICH DAY THIS IS
DAY 1 [ ] 2 [√] 3 [ ] 4 [ ]

Please use a separate line for each item eaten: write in weight of plate; leave a line between different 'plate' entries

A Time eaten am/pm	B TICK A BOX Food eaten at home / away	C TICK A BOX Weighed by mother / other	D Brand name of each item, in full (except for fresh produce)	E Full description of each item including: - whether fresh, frozen, dried, canned - what flavour, whether sweetened - how cooked, what type of fat food fried in	F If fresh fruit or veg, was it home grown? TICK BOX Yes / No	G Weight served gms	H Weight of plate & leftovers gms	TICK ITEMS LEFT OVER	OFFICE USE ONLY Est weight? Tick if YES	Brand	Food	J If any of the item was spilt or eaten by someone else and therefore not reweighed as leftovers TICK BOX - and estimate how much of the original item was lost. Give details of any other problems Yes
8.05am	home [√]1 [ ]2 away	[√]1 [ ]2		Bowl	[ ]1 [ ]2	400	442					[ ]
	[ ]1 [ ]2	[ ]1 [ ]2	Kelloggs	Coco-pops	[ ]1 [ ]2	57	[√]					[ ]
	[ ]1 [ ]2	[ ]1 [ ]2	Unigate	Whole milk, pasteurised, Silver top	[ ]1 [ ]2	63	[√]					[ ]
	[ ]1 [ ]2	[ ]1 [ ]2	Silver Spoon	Sugar (granulated)	[ ]1 [ ]2	6	[√]					[ ]
	[ ]1 [ ]2	[ ]1 [ ]2			[ ]1 [ ]2							[ ]
8.05am	[√]1 [ ]2	[√]1 [ ]2		Glass	[ ]1 [ ]2	220						[ ]
	[ ]1 [ ]2	[ ]1 [ ]2	Tesco	Orange juice, unsweetened longlife	[ ]1 [ ]2	64						[ ]
	[ ]1 [ ]2	[ ]1 [ ]2		diluted with tap water	[ ]1 [ ]2	30						[ ]
	[ ]1 [ ]2	[ ]1 [ ]2			[ ]1 [ ]2							[ ]
11am	[√]1 [ ]2	[√]1 [ ]2		Plate	[ ]1 [ ]2	176						[ ]
	[ ]1 [ ]2	[ ]1 [ ]2	Champion	Sliced softgrain bread, 2 slices toasted	[ ]1 [ ]2	76						[√] ½ slice of toast fed to the dog
	[ ]1 [ ]2	[ ]1 [ ]2	Flora	Margarine	[ ]1 [ ]2	8						[√]
	[ ]1 [ ]2	[ ]1 [ ]2		Marmite	[ ]1 [ ]2	8						[√]
	[ ]1 [ ]2	[ ]1 [ ]2			[ ]1 [ ]2							[ ]

CHECK LIST

EACH PAGE SHOULD HAVE:
day and date;
whether child was well or unwell that day.

WHEN RECORDING:
ALL food should be weighed on a plate and all drinks weighed in a container.

Weigh the plate or container first.

Foods that come in pots or containers and are eaten from them, such as yoghurt, should be weighed before and after contents are eaten.

Start each new food item on a separate line; you can use more than one line to write the description of a food.

Leave a line before starting a new plate or container.

REMEMBER:
Record ALL drinks, including tap water.

Record ALL vitamin and mineral supplements, including fluoride supplements.

Record ALL condiments (eg tomato sauce) used at the table.

Show, by a tick in column F, whether fresh fruit and vegetables were home grown.

Weigh all leftovers on the plate or in the container, and tick those foods which have been left in column H.

Show in column J, whether any of the original item was lost or spilt and could not be reweighed. Estimate the proportion of food or drink lost.

VAAJ/30 1/93

109

Home record diary (E) - recording sheet

110

PLEASE START A NEW PAGE FOR EACH DAY EVEN IF ONLY SOME OF THIS PAGE IS USED

Day .... day   Date

	OFF. USE DAY OF WEEK		TICK A BOX TO SHOW WHETHER CHILD IS WELL OR UNWELL TODAY		Serial Number
			Well 1 Unwell 2		

TICK A BOX TO SHOW WHICH DAY THIS IS
DAY   1   2   3   4

Please use a separate line for each item eaten: write in weight of plate; leave a line between different 'plate' entries

A	B	C		D	E	F		G	H	OFFICE USE ONLY			J
Time eaten am/pm	TICK A BOX Food eaten at away/home	TICK A BOX Weighed by mother/other		Brand name of each item, in full (except for fresh produce)	Full description of each item including: - whether fresh, frozen, dried, canned - what flavour, whether sweetened - how cooked, what type of fat food fried in	If fresh fruit or veg, was it home grown? TICK BOX Yes / No		Weight served gms	Weight of plate & leftovers TICK ITEM	Est weight? Tick if YES	Brand	Food	If any of this item was spilt or eaten by someone else and therefore not reweighed as leftovers TICK BOX - and estimate how much of the original item was lost. Give details of any other problems. → Yes

VA43/3a 1/93

Appendix C

Tables associated with Chapter 5: Data on past use of bottles

Table 1 Use of bottles at night immediately prior to stopping use by children no longer using bottles at the time of interview

Night time use of bottles immediately prior to stopping use	Age when child stopped using bottle		
	Less than 1 year	1-2 years	Over 2 years
	%	%	%
Used every night	13	27	49
Used some nights	6	9	11
Used day only	80	63	39
Base	*284*	*518*	*208*

Table 3 Drinks usually consumed from bottles at night immediately prior to stopping use, by children who had used bottles at night but were no longer doing so at the time of interview

Drinks usually consumed at night	Age when child stopped using bottle		
	Less than 1 year	1-2 years	Over 2 years
	%	%	%
Milk	65	62	61
Water	2	3	2
Drink containing NME sugars	12	19	24
Other drink, not containing NME sugars	9	8	10
Don't know	12	8	4
Base	*57*	*193*	*126*

Table 2 Use of bottles in the day immediately prior to stopping use by children no longer using bottles at the time of interview

Day-time use of bottles immediately prior to stopping use	Age when child stopped using bottle		
	Less than 1 year	1-2 years	Over 2 years
	%	%	%
Used 4 times or more a day	17	14	19
Used 3 times a day	16	12	8
Used 2 times a day	23	16	13
Used once a day	33	35	25
Used less than once a day	4	4	3
Used at night only	7	19	32
Base	*284*	*518*	*208*

Table 4 Drinks usually consumed from bottles during the day immediately prior to stopping use, by children who had used bottles during the day but were no longer doing so at the time of interview

Drinks usually consumed during the day	Age when child stopped using bottle		
	Less than 1 year	1-2 years	Over 2 years
	%	%	%
Milk	66	55	44
Water	1	1	1
Drink containing NME sugars	15	26	37
Other drink, not containing NME sugars	12	12	16
Don't know	6	6	2
Base	*265*	*420*	*142*

Appendix D

Tables associated with Chapter 6: The mean number of teeth with experience of decay in relation to various dental care and dietary behaviour variables

Table 1 The mean number of teeth with any decay experience by age and age started toothbrushing, frequency of toothbrushing and who brushes child's teeth

Age started toothbrushing, frequency of tooth-brushing and who brushes child's teeth	Age of child (in years)							
	$1^1/_2$ - $2^1/_2$		$2^1/_2$ - $3^1/_2$		$3^1/_2$ - $4^1/_2$		All ages	
	Mean	Base	Mean	Base	Mean	Base	Mean	Base
All children	0.1	451	0.5	544	1.3	537	0.6	1532
Age started tooth brushing								
Less than 1 year	0.1	247	0.2	265	0.8	250	0.4	762
1 year to 2 years	0.1	180	0.6	218	1.6	200	0.8	598
Over 2 years	[0]	5	1.1	49	1.7	79	1.4	133
Frequency of tooth brushing								
Less than once a day	0.1	58	0.8	64	2.2	52	1.0	174
Once a day	0	171	0.5	174	1.5	161	0.7	506
More than once a day	0.1	222	0.3	301	1.0	323	0.5	846
Who brushes child's teeth								
Child	0.2	122	0.6	159	1.3	206	*	*
Adult	0.1	140	0.4	124	1.2	100	*	*
Varies - adult or child	0	171	0.4	252	1.2	227	*	*

* This analysis was only carried out for individual age groups.

Table 2 The mean number of teeth with any decay experience by age and child's visits to the dentist, and advice received about dental care

Child's visits to the dentist, and advice received about dental care	Age of child (in years)							
	$1^1/_2$ - $2^1/_2$		$2^1/_2$ - $3^1/_2$		$3^1/_2$ - $4^1/_2$		All ages	
	Mean	Base	Mean	Base	Mean	Base	Mean	Base
All children	0.1	451	0.5	544	1.3	537	0.6	1532
Child's visits to the dentist								
Seen and examined	0.2	110	0.5	286	1.3	413	*	*
Seen not examined	0	43	0.3	44	1.1	20	*	*
Never seen	0.1	297	0.5	211	1.1	103	*	*
Advice about food drink								
Received	0.1	184	0.5	213	1.6	241	0.8	638
Not received	0.1	267	0.5	328	1.0	295	0.5	890
Advice about toothbrushing								
Received	0.1	106	0.3	162	1.5	200	0.8	468
Not received	0.1	345	0.5	379	1.1	336	0.6	1060
Advice to give fluoride supplements								
Received	0.1	98	2.0	121	3.3	129	0.9	348
Not received	0.1	353	1.3	418	2.5	407	0.5	1178
Advice not to give fluoride supplements								
Received	0.1	44	0.2	54	0.6	49	0.3	147
Not received	0.1	407	0.5	486	1.3	486	0.7	1379
Advice on any dental issue								
Received	0	252	0.5	323	1.4	352	0.7	927
Not received	0.2	199	0.5	217	0.9	184	0.5	600

* This analysis was only carried out for individual age groups.

Table 3 The mean number of teeth with any decay experience by age and whether child given fluoride supplements, age started using fluoride supplements, mother's dental attendance pattern and average weekly household expenditure on sweets and chocolates

Use of fluoride supplements, mother's dental attendance pattern and household spending on confectionery	Age of child (in years)							
	1¹/₂ - 2¹/₂		2¹/₂ - 3¹/₂		3¹/₂ - 4¹/₂		All ages	
	Mean	Base	Mean	Base	Mean	Base	Mean	Base
All children	0.1	451	0.5	544	1.3	537	0.6	1532
Whether ever used fluoride supplements								
Used	0.1	72	1.0	98	2.1	111	1.2	281
Never used	0.1	379	0.4	442	1.0	425	0.5	1246
Age started using fluoride supplements								
Less than 1 year	0.1	54	0.7	65	1.7	56	2.5	175
Over 1 year	[0.2]	17	1.6	31	2.6	53	3.4	101
Mother's dental attendance pattern								
Regular	0.1	259	0.3	322	1.0	338	0.5	919
Occasional	0.2	73	0.3	66	1.2	66	0.6	205
Trouble	0.1	109	0.8	142	2.0	121	1.0	372
Average weekly household spending on confectionery								
Less than £2	0.1	250	0.4	280	0.8	282	0.4	812
£2 to £5	0.1	163	0.6	218	1.7	203	0.8	584
More than £5	0.1	37	0.4	42	2.3	50	1.0	129

Table 5 The mean number of teeth with any decay experience by age and night-time drinking practices at the time of interview

Type of night-time drinking practice	Age of child (in years)							
	1¹/₂ - 2¹/₂		2¹/₂ - 3¹/₂		3¹/₂ - 4¹/₂		All ages	
	Mean	Base	Mean	Base	Mean	Base	Mean	Base
All children	0.1	451	0.5	514	1.3	537	0.6	1532
Frequency of drinking in bed								
Every night	0.1	183	0.8	171	1.2	117	0.7	471
Some nights, but not every night	0	52	0.2	89	1.2	118	0.6	259
Never	0.1	216	0.3	281	1.3	301	0.6	798
When drink in bed, type of drink consumed								
Drink containing, non-milk extrinsic sugars	0.2	55	1.2	60	1.8	64	1.1	179
Milk	0.1	103	0.5	87	1.4	47	0.5	237
Water	0	34	0.2	53	0.7	74	0.4	161
If drink in bed every night, usual drink								
Drink containing, non-milk extrinsic sugars	0.3	41	1.7	40	2.0	37	1.3	118
Milk	0.1	90	0.5	68	0.2	31	0.4	189
Vessel usually used when drink at night								
Bottle	0.2	151	0.9	92	2.4	33	*	*
Feeder beaker	0	57	0.7	82	0.5	51	*	*
Mug, cup or glass	[0]	16	0.3	49	1.2	148	*	*

* This analysis was only carried out for individual age groups.

Table 4 The mean number of teeth with any decay experience by age and whether child ever used a bottle, dinky feeder or dummy

Use of bottle, dinky feeder and dummy	Age of child (in years)							
	1¹/₂ - 2¹/₂		2¹/₂ - 3¹/₂		3¹/₂ - 4¹/₂		All ages	
	Mean	Base	Mean	Base	Mean	Base	Mean	Base
All children	0.1	451	0.5	544	1.3	537	0.6	1532
Whether ever used bottle								
Used	0.1	401	0.5	474	1.4	466	0.7	1341
Never used	0.1	50	0.3	67	0.5	70	0.3	187
Whether ever used dinky feeder								
Used	0.1	79	0.4	101	1.4	99	0.6	279
Never used	0.1	372	0.5	440	1.2	437	0.6	1249
Whether ever used dummy								
Used	0.1	252	0.5	282	1.3	287	0.6	821
Never used	0.1	199	0.5	259	1.2	249	0.6	707

Table 6 The mean number of teeth with experience of decay by age and the frequency with which children were reported to consume sugar confectionery, chocolate confectionery, biscuits, cakes and ice cream or ice lollies (from the dietary interview)

Food frequency data

Frequency of consuming sugar confectionery, chocolate confectionery, biscuits, cakes and ice creams or ice lollies	Age of child (in years)					
	1½ - 2½		2½ - 3½		3½ - 4½	
	Mean	*Base*	Mean	*Base*	Mean	*Base*
Mean number of teeth with experience of decay for all children	0.1	*451*	0.5	*514*	1.3	*537*
Sugar confectionery						
Most days or more often	0.1	*147*	0.6	*254*	1.7	*255*
Less frequently than most days*	0.1	*304*	0.3	*289*	0.8	*281*
Chocolate confectionery						
Once a day or more often	0.1	*64*	0.5	*100*	1.2	*93*
Most days	0	*87*	0.4	*136*	1.7	*110*
At least once a week	0.1	*228*	0.4	*247*	1.0	*260*
Less frequently than at least once a week*	0	*70*	0.6	*60*	1.5	*73*
Biscuits						
More than once a day	0.3	*93*	0.6	*114*	1.0	*115*
Once a day	0.1	*103*	0.5	*118*	1.3	*108*
Most days	0	*166*	0.5	*204*	1.3	*209*
Less frequently than most days*	0	*87*	0.4	*108*	1.3	*105*
Cakes						
Most days or more often	0	*53*	0.6	*85*	1.2	*81*
At least once a week	0.1	*243*	0.5	*306*	1.2	*300*
At least once a month	0.1	*91*	0.5	*100*	1.6	*97*
Less than once a month*	0.1	*64*	0.3	*52*	1.0	*58*
Ice cream or ice lollies						
Most days or more often	0.1	*147*	0.6	*254*	1.7	*255*
At least once a week	0.1	*154*	0.3	*181*	0.8	*219*
At least once a month	0.1	*37*	0.4	*48*	[0.6]	*29*
Less than once a month*	0	*113*	0.3	*60*	1.2	*33*

* Including non-consumers.

Table 7 The mean number of teeth with experience of decay by age and the frequency with which children were reported to consume carbonated drinks*, blackcurrant drinks† and fruit juice (from the dietary interview)

Food frequency data

Frequency of consuming carbonated drinks, blackcurrant drinks and fruit juice	Age of child (in years)					
	1½ - 2½		2½ - 3½		3½ - 4½	
	Mean	*Base*	Mean	*Base*	Mean	*Base*
Mean number of teeth with experience of decay for all children	0.1	*451*	0.5	*514*	1.3	*537*
Carbonated drinks*						
Most days or more often	0.1	*75*	0.9	*143*	1.8	*157*
Less often than most days§	0.1	*376*	0.3	*400*	1.0	*379*
Blackcurrant drinks†						
More than once a day	0.1	*64*	0.5	*80*	0.7	*84*
Once a day or most days	0.1	*63*	0.9	*83*	1.1	*87*
At least once a week	0	*45*	0.4	*60*	1.5	*66*
Sometimes but less frequently than at least once a week	0.1	*78*	0.3	*98*	1.2	*117*
Never	0.1	*200*	0.4	*222*	1.6	*183*
Fruit juice						
Once a day or more often	0.1	*92*	0.4	*113*	0.8	*95*
Most days	0	*64*	0.6	*78*	1.1	*71*
At least once a week	0	*81*	0.5	*109*	1.1	*122*
At least once a month	0.1	*54*	0.2	*59*	1.6	*70*
Less than once a month	0	*32*	0.2	*43*	1.3	*43*
Never	0.2	*128*	0.7	*142*	1.7	*134*

* Including diet carbonated drinks, but excluding mineral water.
† Including diet blackcurrant drinks.
§ Including non-consumers.

Table 8 The mean number of teeth with any decay experience according to the frequency of consumption of selected foods containing sugars and the average daily intake of these foods and selected nutrients, by age of child; data presented for those with intakes below the 10th percentile value and above the 90th percentile value

Weighed intake data

Frequency of consumption and average intakes of foods containing sugars and selected nutrients	Age of child (in years) and percentile											
	1½ - 2½				2½ - 3½				3½ - 4½			
	10		90		10		90		10		90	
	Mean	*Base*	Mean	*Base*	Mean	*Base*	Mean	*Base*	Mean	*Base*	Mean	*Base*
Average daily frequency of consumption of:												
Sugar confectionery	0.1	*233*	0.2	*41*	0.5	*183*	0.8	*32*	1.2	*174*	1.3	*44*
Chocolate confectionery	0	*123*	0	*40*	0.8	*116*	0.7	*42*	1.6	*133*	1.6	*50*
Soft drinks*	0.1	*85*	0.1	*42*	0.6	*67*	0.5	*51*	1.2	*54*	0.8	*50*
Fruit juice	0.1	*276*	0	*37*	0.5	*338*	0.1	*48*	1.5	*325*	0.4	*46*
Various foods containing sugars†	0	*45*	0.1	*42*	0.7	*59*	0.5	*48*	1.2	*51*	0.9	*50*
Average daily intake in grams§ of:												
Sugar confectionery	0.1	*233*	0.2	*41*	0.5	*183*	0.8	*48*	1.2	*174*	1.3	*52*
Chocolate confectionery	0	*123*	0.1	*43*	0.8	*116*	0.6	*51*	1.6	*133*	1.1	*52*
Soft drinks*	0.1	*85*	0	*41*	0.6	*67*	0.7	*51*	1.2	*54*	0.7	*52*
Fruit juice	0.1	*276*	0	*38*	0.5	*338*	0.2	*48*	1.5	*325*	0.3	*51*
Various foods containing sugars†	0	*41*	0	*38*	0.8	*56*	0.7	*52*	1.6	*50*	0.6	*52*
Average daily intake in grams of:**												
Total sugars	0	*44*	0	*37*	0.7	*52*	0.6	*53*	1.7	*52*	1.3	*52*
Non-milk extrinsic sugars	0	*42*	0.1	*38*	0.8	*52*	0.4	*52*	1.4	*52*	0.9	*52*
Intrinsic and milk sugars and starch	0.2	*45*	0.1	*40*	0.8	*49*	0.5	*51*	1.9	*52*	1.7	*52*
Carbohydrate	0	*43*	0	*39*	1.0	*49*	0.4	*53*	1.7	*52*	1.1	*51*

* Includes fruit squashes with sugar, and carbonated drinks.
† Includes intakes from the following food groups: biscuits; buns, cakes, pastries; fruit pies; milk, sponge and other puddings; ice cream; yogurt; fruit in syrup; sugar; preserves; sugar confectionery; chocolate confectionery; fruit juice; other soft drinks.
§ Weight of sugary products consumed.
** Nutrient variable measuring actual intake of sugars/nutrients within all foods, including intakes from dietary supplements.

Appendix E Tables associated with Chapter 7: The proportion of children with erosion in relation to various background and behavioural characteristics

Table 1 Proportion of children with erosion, by age and social class of the head of household

Social class of head of household	Age of child (in years)			
	$1^1/_2$ - $2^1/_2$	$2^1/_2$ - $3^1/_2$	$3^1/_2$ - $4^1/_2$	All ages
	Percentage of children with each type of erosion			
Non-manual				
Any buccal erosion	10	10	9	10
Buccal erosion into dentine or pulp	2	2	3	2
Any palatal erosion	12	20	26	20
Palatal erosion into dentine or pulp	4	6	12	7
*Bases**	*205/200*	*242/237*	*224/224*	*671/661*
Manual				
Any buccal erosion	3	9	17	10
Buccal erosion into dentine or pulp	1	2	3	2
Any palatal erosion	7	17	30	19
Palatal erosion into dentine or pulp	2	7	13	8
*Bases**	*237/225*	*282/275*	*273/276*	*792/776*

* Children with full examinations for buccal/palatal erosion.

Table 2 Proportion of children with erosion, by age and mother's highest educational qualification

Mother's highest educational qualification	Age of child (in years)			
	$1^1/_2$ - $2^1/_2$	$2^1/_2$ - $3^1/_2$	$3^1/_2$ - $4^1/_2$	All ages
	Percentage of children with each type of erosion			
GCE 'A' level or above				
Any buccal erosion	8	11	14	11
Buccal erosion into dentine or pulp	0	1	3	1
Any palatal erosion	10	18	30	19
Palatal erosion into dentine or pulp	3	5	10	6
*Bases**	*140/135*	*152/147*	*146/146*	*438/428*
Other				
Any buccal erosion	6	9	15	10
Buccal erosion into dentine or pulp	1	3	3	2
Any palatal erosion	8	21	31	20
Palatal erosion into dentine or pulp	3	8	15	9
*Bases**	*237/230*	*264/256*	*244/246*	*745/732*
No qualification				
Any buccal erosion	8	12	12	11
Buccal erosion into dentine or pulp	4	3	3	3
Any palatal erosion	10	15	24	17
Palatal erosion into dentine or pulp	5	4	12	7
*Bases**	*85/80*	*125/126*	*122/123*	*332/329*

* Children with full examinations for buccal/palatal erosion.

Table 3 Proportion of children with erosion, by age and whether parents in receipt of Income Support or Family Credit

Whether parents in receipt of Income Support or Family Credit (benefits)	Age of child (in years)			
	$1^1/_2$ - $2^1/_2$	$2^1/_2$ - $3^1/_2$	$3^1/_2$ - $4^1/_2$	All ages
	Percentage of children with each type of erosion			
Receiving benefits				
Any buccal erosion	8	11	16	12
Buccal erosion into dentine or pulp	4	3	5	4
Any palatal erosion	12	17	31	21
Palatal erosion into dentine or pulp	4	6	14	8
*Bases**	*143/137*	*175/170*	*153/156*	*471/463*
Not receiving benefits				
Any buccal erosion	7	9	13	10
Buccal erosion into dentine or pulp	0	2	2	1
Any palatal erosion	8	19	28	19
Palatal erosion into dentine or pulp	3	6	13	8
*Bases**	*319/308*	*367/360*	*360/360*	*1046/1028*

* Children with full examinations for buccal/palatal erosion.

Table 4 Proportion of children with erosion, by age and region

Region	Age of child (in years)			
	$1^1/_2$ - $2^1/_2$	$2^1/_2$ - $3^1/_2$	$3^1/_2$ - $4^1/_2$	All ages
	Percentage of children with each type of erosion			
Scotland				
Any buccal erosion	3	19	26	18
Buccal erosion into dentine or pulp	0	2	3	2
Any palatal erosion	3	31	34	25
Palatal erosion into dentine or pulp	0	11	12	9
*Bases**	*38/ 36*	*47/ 45*	*58/ 58*	*143/139*
North				
Any buccal erosion	11	11	14	12
Buccal erosion into dentine or pulp	4	3	4	4
Any palatal erosion	16	22	35	24
Palatal erosion into dentine or pulp	7	12	22	14
*Bases**	*108/100*	*147/141*	*111/111*	*366/352*
Central, South West and Wales				
Any buccal erosion	4	5	13	7
Buccal erosion into dentine or pulp	1	1	3	1
Any palatal erosion	6	12	23	14
Palatal erosion into dentine or pulp	2	0	9	4
*Bases**	*164/160*	*188/186*	*178/179*	*530/525*
London and the South East				
Any buccal erosion	9	12	11	11
Buccal erosion into dentine or pulp	1	3	2	2
Any palatal erosion	10	19	30	20
Palatal erosion into dentine or pulp	3	6	12	7
*Bases**	*152/149*	*160/158*	*167/169*	*479/476*

* Children with full examinations for buccal/palatal erosion.

Table 5 Proportion of children with erosion, by age and age when started toothbrushing

Age when started toothbrushing	Age of child (in years)			
	$1^1/_2$ - $2^1/_2$	$2^1/_2$ - $3^1/_2$	$3^1/_2$ - $4^1/_2$	All ages
	Percentage of children with each type of erosion			
Less than one year				
Any buccal erosion	9	9	12	10
Buccal erosion into dentine or pulp	1	2	2	2
Any palatal erosion	10	21	27	19
Palatal erosion into dentine or pulp	4	7	13	8
*Bases**	*252/244*	*262/256*	*240/241*	*754/741*
One year to two years				
Any buccal erosion	5	11	16	11
Buccal erosion into dentine or pulp	2	3	4	3
Any palatal erosion	7	15	34	19
Palatal erosion into dentine or pulp	2	6	13	7
*Bases**	*187/179*	*221/216*	*192/194*	*600/589*
Over two years				
Any buccal erosion	[0]	10	15	13
Buccal erosion into dentine or pulp	[0]	2	1	2
Any palatal erosion	[0]	16	24	20
Palatal erosion into dentine or pulp	[0]	2	12	8
*Bases**	*5/ 5*	*49/ 49*	*74/ 74*	*128/128*

* Children with full examinations for buccal/palatal erosion.

Table 6 Proportion of children with erosion, by age and frequency of toothbrushing

Frequency of toothbrushing	Age of child (in years)			
	$1^1/_2$ - $2^1/_2$	$2^1/_2$ - $3^1/_2$	$3^1/_2$ - $4^1/_2$	All ages
	Percentage of children with each type of erosion			
Less than once a day				
Any buccal erosion	8	11	16	11
Buccal erosion into dentine or pulp	2	5	6	4
Any palatal erosion	12	14	35	19
Palatal erosion into dentine or pulp	7	5	16	9
*Bases**	*63/ 59*	*66/ 65*	*50/ 51*	*179/175*
Once a day				
Any buccal erosion	6	9	17	10
Buccal erosion into dentine or pulp	1	1	3	2
Any palatal erosion	7	21	30	19
Palatal erosion into dentine or pulp	2	8	14	8
*Bases**	*178/174*	*172/167*	*151/152*	*501/493*
More than once a day				
Any buccal erosion	8	10	12	10
Buccal erosion into dentine or pulp	1	2	3	2
Any palatal erosion	10	18	27	20
Palatal erosion into dentine or pulp	3	6	12	8
*Bases**	*221/212*	*302/296*	*313/314*	*836/822*

* Children with full examinations for buccal/palatal erosion.

Table 7 Proportion of children with erosion, by age and who brushes child's teeth

Who brushes teeth	Age of child (in years)		
	$1^1/_2 - 2^1/_2$	$2^1/_2 - 3^1/_2$	$3^1/_2 - 4^1/_2$
	Percentage of children with each type of erosion		
Child			
Any buccal erosion	6	12	15
Buccal erosion into dentine or pulp	2	1	3
Any palatal erosion	8	18	31
Palatal erosion into dentine or pulp	3	5	16
*Bases**	*120/116*	*158/152*	*196/197*
Adult			
Any buccal erosion	8	11	11
Buccal erosion into dentine or pulp	1	5	3
Any palatal erosion	10	20	26
Palatal erosion into dentine or pulp	5	8	7
*Bases**	*146/143*	*125/123*	*96/ 96*
Child or adult - varies			
Any buccal erosion	7	8	14
Buccal erosion into dentine or pulp	-	2	3
Any palatal erosion	8	18	29
Palatal erosion into dentine or pulp	1	6	13
*Bases**	*179/170*	*252/249*	*219/221*

* Children with full examinations for buccal/palatal erosion.

Table 9 Proportion of children with erosion, by age and whether ever used a bottle

Whether used a bottle	Age of child (in years)			
	$1^1/_2 - 2^1/_2$	$2^1/_2 - 3^1/_2$	$3^1/_2 - 4^1/_2$	All ages
	Percentage of children with each type of erosion			
Used a bottle				
Any buccal erosion	7	10	14	11
Buccal erosion into dentine or pulp	1	3	3	2
Any palatal erosion	9	19	28	19
Palatal erosion into dentine or pulp	3	6	12	7
*Bases**	*410/395*	*473/462*	*445/448*	*1328/1305*
Never used a bottle				
Any buccal erosion	6	7	10	8
Buccal erosion into dentine or pulp	2	0	3	2
Any palatal erosion	8	15	33	20
Palatal erosion into dentine or pulp	4	6	17	10
*Bases**	*52/ 50*	*69/ 68*	*69/ 69*	*190/187*

* Children with full examinations for buccal/palatal erosion.

Table 8 Proportion of children with erosion, by age and whether ever used fluoride supplements

Whether used fluoride supplements	Age of child (in years)			
	$1^1/_2 - 2^1/_2$	$2^1/_2 - 3^1/_2$	$3^1/_2 - 4^1/_2$	All ages
	Percentage of children with each type of erosion			
Used fluoride supplements				
Any buccal erosion	7	14	15	12
Buccal erosion into dentine or pulp	-	1	5	2
Any palatal erosion	9	25	31	23
Palatal erosion into dentine or pulp	3	10	16	10
*Bases**	*71/ 69*	*96/ 92*	*102/103*	*269/264*
Never used fluoride supplements				
Any buccal erosion	7	9	14	10
Buccal erosion into dentine or pulp	2	2	2	2
Any palatal erosion	9	17	29	19
Palatal erosion into dentine or pulp	3	5	12	7
*Bases**	*391/376*	*445/437*	*412/414*	*1248/1227*

* Children with full examinations for buccal/palatal erosion.

Table 10 Proportion of children with erosion, by age and whether ever used a dinky feeder

Whether used a dinky feeder	Age of child (in years)			
	$1^1/_2 - 2^1/_2$	$2^1/_2 - 3^1/_2$	$3^1/_2 - 4^1/_2$	All ages
	Percentage of children with each type of erosion			
Used a dinky feeder				
Any buccal erosion	6	9	19	12
Buccal erosion into dentine or pulp	1	2	2	2
Any palatal erosion	7	20	35	22
Palatal erosion into dentine or pulp	3	3	11	6
*Bases**	*78/ 73*	*100/ 98*	*93/ 94*	*271/265*
Never used a dinky feeder				
Any buccal erosion	7	10	13	10
Buccal erosion into dentine or pulp	1	2	3	2
Any palatal erosion	10	18	28	19
Palatal erosion into dentine or pulp	3	7	14	8
*Bases**	*384/372*	*442/432*	*421/423*	*1247/1227*

* Children with full examinations for buccal/palatal erosion.

Table 11   Proportion of children with erosion, by age and whether child ever used a dummy

Whether used a dummy	Age of child (in years)			
	$1^1/_2$ - $2^1/_2$	$2^1/_2$ - $3^1/_2$	$3^1/_2$ - $4^1/_2$	All ages
	Percentage of children with each type of erosion			
Used a dummy				
Any buccal erosion	5	9	16	11
Buccal erosion into dentine or pulp	2	1	3	2
Any palatal erosion	8	18	27	18
Palatal erosion into dentine or pulp	2	4	10	6
*Bases**	*257/245*	*279/275*	*276/277*	*812/797*
Never used a dummy				
Any buccal erosion	9	11	11	10
Buccal erosion into dentine or pulp	1	3	3	2
Any palatal erosion	11	20	31	21
Palatal erosion into dentine or pulp	4	8	17	10
*Bases**	*205/200*	*263/255*	*238/240*	*706/695*

* Children with full examinations for buccal/palatal erosion.

Table 12   Proportion of children with erosion, by age and average weekly household spending on chocolates and sweets

Average weekly household spending on chocolates and sweets	Age of child (in years)			
	$1^1/_2$ - $2^1/_2$	$2^1/_2$ - $3^1/_2$	$3^1/_2$ - $4^1/_2$	All ages
	Percentage of children with each type of erosion			
Less than £2 a week				
Any buccal erosion	5	10	11	9
Buccal erosion into dentine or pulp	-	3	1	1
Any palatal erosion	8	19	29	19
Palatal erosion into dentine or pulp	1	6	12	7
*Bases**	*256/247*	*282/276*	*270/271*	*808/794*
£2 to £5 a week				
Any buccal erosion	9	10	16	12
Buccal erosion into dentine or pulp	3	1	4	3
Any palatal erosion	9	19	29	20
Palatal erosion into dentine or pulp	6	7	14	9
*Bases**	*169/161*	*217/212*	*193/196*	*579/569*
Over £5 a week				
Any buccal erosion	11	10	20	14
Buccal erosion into dentine or pulp	3	2	6	4
Any palatal erosion	17	12	33	21
Palatal erosion into dentine or pulp	6	2	16	9
*Bases**	*36/ 36*	*42/41*	*50/ 49*	*128/126*

* Children with full examinations for buccal/palatal erosion.

Table 13   Proportion of children with erosion, by age and frequency of consuming sugar confectionery

Food frequency data

Frequency of consuming sugar confectionery	Age of child (in years)		
	$1^1/_2$ - $2^1/_2$	$2^1/_2$ - $3^1/_2$	$3^1/_2$ - $4^1/_2$
	Percentage of children with each type of erosion		
At least most days of the week			
Any buccal erosion	7	11	16
Buccal erosion into dentine or pulp	3	4	4
Any palatal erosion	9	21	32
Palatal erosion into dentine or pulp	4	7	15
*Bases**	*148/139*	*252/246*	*239/240*
Less frequently than above			
Any buccal erosion	7	9	12
Buccal erosion into dentine or pulp	0	1	2
Any palatal erosion	10	16	26
Palatal erosion into dentine or pulp	3	5	12
*Bases**	*314/306*	*289/283*	*274/276*

* Children with full examinations for buccal/palatal erosion.

Table 14   Proportion of children with erosion, by age and frequency of consuming carbonated drinks

Food frequency data

Frequency of consuming carbonated drinks (including low calorie carbonated drinks)	Age of child (in years)		
	$1^1/_2$ - $2^1/_2$	$2^1/_2$ - $3^1/_2$	$3^1/_2$ - $4^1/_2$
	Percentage of children with each type of erosion		
At least most days of the week			
Any buccal erosion	7	11	19
Buccal erosion into dentine or pulp	3	4	3
Any palatal erosion	9	22	32
Palatal erosion into dentine or pulp	3	10	16
*Bases**	*75/ 70*	*139/134*	*146/146*
Less frequently than above			
Any buccal erosion	7	10	12
Buccal erosion into dentine or pulp	1	1	3
Any palatal erosion	9	17	28
Palatal erosion into dentine or pulp	3	5	12
*Bases**	*387/375*	*403/396*	*367/370*

* Children with full examinations for buccal/palatal erosion .

Table 15 Proportion of children with erosion, by age and frequency of having a drink in bed (at time of interview)

Frequency of having a drink in bed	Age of child (in years)			
	1½ - 2½	2½ - 3½	3½ - 4½	All ages
	Percentage of children with each type of erosion			
Every night				
Any buccal erosion	8	10	13	10
Buccal erosion into dentine or pulp	2	4	5	3
Any palatal erosion	12	17	29	18
Palatal erosion into dentine or pulp	4	7	13	8
*Bases**	*185/179*	*171/167*	*109/109*	*465/455*
Some nights				
Any buccal erosion	6	9	12	9
Buccal erosion into dentine or pulp	-	2	1	1
Any palatal erosion	4	20	31	22
Palatal erosion into dentine or pulp	2	5	10	7
*Bases**	*54/ 51*	*89/ 87*	*113/115*	*256/253*
Never				
Any buccal erosion	7	10	15	11
Buccal erosion into dentine or pulp	1	1	3	2
Any palatal erosion	8	19	28	19
Palatal erosion into dentine or pulp	2	6	14	8
*Bases**	*223/215*	*282/276*	*292/293*	*797/784*

* Children with full examinations for buccal/palatal erosion.

Table 16 Proportion of children with erosion, by age and vessel used when having a drink in bed

Vessel used when having a drink in bed	Age of child (in years)		
	1½ - 2½	2½ - 3½	3½ - 4½
	Percentage of children with each type of erosion		
Bottle			
Any buccal erosion	9	13	3
Buccal erosion into dentine or pulp	2	5	3
Any palatal erosion	13	19	20
Palatal erosion into dentine or pulp	5	9	3
*Bases**	*154/148*	*94/ 90*	*30/ 30*
Feeder beaker			
Any buccal erosion	5	6	11
Buccal erosion into dentine or pulp	0	0	2
Any palatal erosion	7	21	34
Palatal erosion into dentine or pulp	-	7	9
*Bases**	*57/ 57*	*83/ 81*	*47/ 47*
Mug, cup or glass			
Any buccal erosion	[0]	11	14
Buccal erosion into dentine or pulp	[0]	5	3
Any palatal erosion	[0]	13	31
Palatal erosion into dentine or pulp	[0]	3	15
*Bases**	*16/ 13*	*76/ 76*	*142/144*

* Children with full examinations for buccal/palatal erosion.

Table 17 Proportion of children with erosion, by age and drink usually had when drinking in bed

Usual drink when drinking in bed	Age of child (in years)			
	1½ - 2½	2½ - 3½	3½ - 4½	All ages
	Percentage of children with each type of erosion			
Milk				
Any buccal erosion	5	11	5	7
Buccal erosion into dentine or pulp	-	5	-	2
Any palatal erosion	8	17	24	14
Palatal erosion into dentine or pulp	2	6	7	4
*Bases**	*108/104*	*88/ 84*	*43/ 45*	*239/233*
Water				
Any buccal erosion	6	10	11	10
Buccal erosion into dentine or pulp	-	2	1	1
Any palatal erosion	7	13	27	19
Palatal erosion into dentine or pulp	0	2	11	6
*Bases**	*32/ 30*	*52/ 52*	*73/ 73*	*157/155*
Drink containing NME sugars				
Any buccal erosion	12	10	20	14
Buccal erosion into dentine or pulp	4	5	7	5
Any palatal erosion	11	21	41	24
Palatal erosion into dentine or pulp	5	9	17	11
*Bases**	*57/ 56*	*59/ 57*	*59/ 59*	*175/172*
Other drink, not containing NME sugars				
Any buccal erosion	12	8	11	10
Buccal erosion into dentine or pulp	3	2	2	2
Any palatal erosion	26	21	30	25
Palatal erosion into dentine or pulp	13	10	11	11
*Bases**	*33/ 31*	*52/ 52*	*44/ 44*	*129/127*

* Children with full examinations for buccal/palatal erosion.

Table 18 Proportion of children with any buccal erosion into dentine or pulp for children whose average daily frequency of consumption and intakes of certain foods and nutrients, were below the 10th percentile value and above the 90th percentile value, by age

Weighed intake data

Frequency of consumption of selected foods containing sugars and average intakes of these foods and selected nutrients	Age of child (in years) and percentile											
	1½ - 2½				2½ - 3½				3½ - 4½			
	10		90		10		90		10		90	
	%	base	%	base	%	base	%	base	%	base	%	base
Average daily frequency of consumption of:												
Sugar confectionery	1	241	-	43	3	185	-	30	2	169	2	41
Chocolate confectionery	-	125	-	41	5	118	2	42	1	121	6	47
Soft drinks*	-	86	5	44	3	66	2	50	2	51	6	47
Fruit juice	1	279	-	39	3	334	-	48	4	312	2	45
Various foods containing sugars†	-	44	2	44	5	60	-	46	2	50	4	50
Average daily intake in grams§ of:												
Sugar confectionery	1	241	-	43	3	185	7	46	2	169	6	50
Chocolate confectionery	-	125	-	44	5	118	4	49	1	121	4	48
Soft drinks*	-	86	5	43	3	66	4	50	2	51	4	50
Fruit juice	1	279	-	42	3	334	-	48	4	312	-	50
Various foods containing sugars†	-	44	5	42	5	55	4	52	2	49	4	50
Average daily intake in grams of:**												
Total sugars	-	44	-	40	6	51	-	51	2	52	6	50
Non-milk extrinsic sugars	0	43	2	42	6	52	0	48	2	50	6	50
Intrinsic and milk sugars and starch	7	44	-	39	4	49	2	52	-	46	2	48
Carbohydrate	-	43	-	40	6	49	-	51	2	49	6	49

* Includes fruit squashes with sugar, and carbonated drinks.

† Includes intakes from the following food groups: biscuits; buns, cakes, pastries; fruit pies; milk, sponge and other puddings; ice cream; yogurt; fruit in syrup; sugar; preserves; sugar confectionery; chocolate confectionery; fruit juice; other soft drinks.

§ Weight of products containing sugars consumed.

** Nutrient variable measuring actual intake of sugars/nutrients within all foods, including intakes from dietary supplements.

Table 19 Proportion of children with any palatal erosion into dentine or pulp for children whose average daily frequency of consumption and intakes of certain foods and nutrients, were below the 10th percentile value and above the 90th percentile value, by age

Weighed intake data

Frequency of consumption of selected foods containing sugars and average intakes of those foods and selected nutrients	Age of child (in years) and percentile											
	½ - 2½				2½ - 3½				3½ - 4½			
	10		90		10		90		10		90	
	%	base	%	base	%	base	%	base	%	base	%	base
Average daily frequency of consumption of:												
Sugar confectionery	3	230	2	43	3	179	3	31	13	170	5	41
Chocolate confectionery	-	118	7	41	7	115	7	41	14	124	17	47
Soft drinks*	2	82	10	42	3	65	8	50	4	51	12	48
Fruit juice	4	270	-	37	6	327	4	48	15	315	9	45
Various foods containing sugars†	-	41	5	42	6	54	4	46	6	50	18	50
Average daily intake in grams§ of												
Sugar confectionery	3	230	-	43	3	179	15	47	13	170	18	50
Chocolate confectionery	-	118	9	44	7	115	10	49	14	124	10	48
Soft drinks*	2	82	10	42	3	65	10	50	4	51	20	50
Fruit juice	4	270	-	41	6	327	4	48	15	315	10	50
Various foods containing sugars†	-	42	10	42	2	53	8	52	6	49	24	50
Average daily intake in grams of:**												
Total sugars	-	43	5	40	2	50	2	51	17	53	20	50
Non-milk extrinsic sugars	-	40	5	41	4	50	4	48	12	51	20	50
Intrinsic and milk sugars and starch	12	43	5	38	6	47	10	52	19	47	15	48
Carbohydrate	2	43	5	40	2	48	-	51	12	50	20	49

* Includes fruit squashes with sugar and carbonated drinks, including low-calorie carbonated drinks.

† Includes intakes from the following food groups: biscuits; buns, cakes, pastries; fruit pies; milk, sponge and other puddings; ice cream; yogurt; fruit in syrup; sugar; preserves; sugar confectionery; chocolate confectionery; fruit juice; other soft drinks.

§ Weight of products containing sugars consumed.

** Nutrient variable measuring actual intake of sugars/nutrients within all foods, including intakes from dietary supplements.

Appendix F   Sampling errors

This appendix briefly explains the sources of error associated with survey estimates and presents the sampling errors and design factors for a number of key variables shown in this Report. More detailed information about sampling errors and design factors, and the sampling errors and design factors for a wider range of variables can be found in Appendix D of the Diet and Nutrition Survey Report.[1]

Sources of error

Survey results are subject to various sources of error; these are usually referred to as random and systematic errors. The total error in a survey estimate is the difference between the estimate derived from the data collected and the true value for the population.

Random error

Random error is the part of total error that would be expected to average zero if a number of repeats of the same survey were carried out based on different samples from the population. Sampling error is an important component of random error, arising because estimates are based on a sample rather than a census of the population. The size of the sample and the sample design influence the magnitude of sampling error. Random error may also arise from other sources such as the informant's interpretation of the questions or from errors associated with taking measurements. As with all surveys carried out by Social Survey Division, considerable efforts were made on this survey to minimise sampling error through careful sample design and non-sampling random error through interviewer and dentist training.

Systematic error

Systematic errors are those which would not be expected to average to zero over repeats of the survey, for example biases due to the omission of certain parts of the population from the sampling frame and bias from interviewer or coder variation. Non-response bias is another type of systematic error which occurs if non-respondents to the survey or to particular elements of the survey differ in some respects from respondents, so that the responding sample is not representative of the total population. Non-response can be minimised by training interviewers in how to deal with potential refusals, and with strategies to minimise non-contacts. However a certain level of non-response is inevitable in any voluntary survey. Chapter 2 showed that the age profile of the dental sample was slightly different to that of the diet and nutrition survey due to greater non-response among younger children to the later elements of the survey; non-response bias was not found for other characteristics of the sample such as social class or region.

Standard errors and design factors

In considering the reliability of survey estimates, standard errors are often used. These assess errors associated with the sample design; they cannot take account of other potential errors such as non-response bias, or random error due to misunderstanding of questions. Standard errors are generally calculated on the assumption of a simple random sample design and therefore need to be adjusted for the effect of a complex sample design. As described in Chapters 1 and 2 this survey used a multi-stage sample design which involved both clustering (using postcode sectors as primary sampling units, PSUs) and stratification. Clustering is likely to increase standard errors while stratification tends to reduce them. Social Survey Division uses a software program called EPSILON[2] to calculate the true standard errors associated with survey estimates and to produce design factors. Design factors can be used as multipliers when conducting significance tests which are based on the assumption of a simple random sample design, to adjust for the complex design of a particular sample. In this Report tests for significant differences between survey means generally used true standard errors and the design factor was used as a multiplier in testing differences between proportions. In some cases where data were analysed by subgroups, the exact design factors were not calculated and conservative design factors were estimated. The formulae used to test for significant differences were:

For proportions:

$$\sqrt{\frac{(p_1 \; q_1)}{n_1} + \frac{(p_2 \; q_2)}{n_2}} \times 1.96 \times \textit{deft}$$

where p_1 and p_2 are the observed percentages for the two subsamples, q_1 and q_2 are respectively $(100-p_1)$ and $(100-p_2)$, and n_1 and n_2 are the subsample sizes. The value of 1.96 is used to test for significant differences at the 95% level ($p<0.05$); a value of 2.58 is used to test for significant differences at the 99% level.[3]

For means:

$$\sqrt{se_1^2 + se_2^2} \times 1.96$$

Where se_1 and se_2 are the true standard errors of two means.[4]

Tables 1 to 8 present the true standard errors and design factors for some of the key variables presented in this Report. The size of the design factor varies between survey variables reflecting the degree to which a characteristic is clustered within PSUs, or is distributed between strata. For a single variable the size of the design factor also varies according to the size of the subgroup on which the estimate is based, and on the distribution of the subgroup between PSUs and strata. Design factors below 1.0 show that the complex sample design improved on the estimate that would be expected from a simple random sample, probably due to the benefits of stratification; design factors greater than 1.0 show a less reliable estimate than might be gained from a simple random sample, due to the effects of clustering.

Over 80% of the design factors calculated for estimates from this survey were less than 1.2; design factors of this order are considered to be small and indicate that a characteristic is not markedly clustered geographically.

For the socio-demographic characteristics where geographic clustering would be expected, design factors above 1.2 were found for virtually all characteristics (Table 1). From Table 1 it can be seen that where a variable has only two categories representing 100% of responses, for example whether a child's parents were or were not receiving Income Support or Family Credit, the standard errors and design factors are the same for both responses. In subsequent tables only one aspect of such variables will be considered, for example in Table 2 standard errors and design factors are shown only for children with experience of caries although the same design factors relate to those with no experience of caries.

With the exception of some of the design factors for erosion, low standard errors and design factors were found for all aspects of the dental examination (Table 2). The design factors for treated caries (fillings and extractions), and for trauma of the incisors, were below 1.1 in all cases, while those for active caries were slightly higher although still below 1.2 within each age cohort. Higher design factors were found for the measures of erosion into the enamel, dentine or pulp (from 1.2 to 2.2). When the erosion data were presented in Chapter 7 attention was drawn to the possibility of high levels of examiner variability. The high design factors for 'any buccal erosion' and 'any palatal erosion' highlight this examiner variation. The design factors for erosion into the dentine or pulp only, were of a similar order to those for other aspects of the dental examination.

Design factors for data from the dental questionnaire, the dietary questionnaire and the four-day weighed intake diary were rarely above 1.2, and were generally between 0.9 and 1.2. Tables 3 to 8 show the standard errors and design factors for a selection of those variables for which calculations were carried out.

Table 1 True standard errors and design factors for socio-demographic characteristics of the dental sample

Characteristic	% (p)	Standard error of p	Design factor
Age			
1½ to 2½ years	29.98	1.08	0.96
2½ to 3½ years	36.24	1.13	0.96
3½ to 4½ years	33.78	1.08	0.93
Region			
Scotland	9.89	0.85	1.16
Northern	24.85	1.24	1.17
Central, South West and Wales	34.20	1.45	1.24
London and South East	31.06	1.47	1.29
Social class of head of household			
Non-manual	46.50	1.64	1.31
Manual	53.50	1.64	1.31
Highest educational qualification of child's mother			
GCE 'A' Level or higher	29.06	1.77	1.58
Other	49.49	1.52	1.24
No qualification	21.45	1.48	1.47
Employment status of head of household			
Working	75.09	1.60	1.51
Unemployed	9.83	0.77	1.05
Economically inactive	15.08	1.35	1.54
Family type			
Couple with child/children	82.38	1.25	1.33
Lone-parent family	17.62	1.25	1.33
Whether child's parents in receipt of Income Support or Family Credit			
Receiving benefit(s)	31.56	1.77	1.55
Not receiving benefit(s)	68.44	1.77	1.55
Sample size	*1658*	*1658*	*1658*

Table 2 Proportion of children with different dental conditions and the associated standard errors and design factors

Measure from examination	Percentage of children with characteristic % p	Sample size	Standard error of p	Design factor
Experience of caries				
1^1/$_2$ to 2^1/$_2$ years	3.99	451	1.05	1.14
2^1/$_2$ to 3^1/$_2$ years	13.97	544	1.55	1.04
3^1/$_2$ to 4^1/$_2$ years	30.17	537	2.25	1.13
All children	16.71	1532	1.11	1.17
Any active decay				
1^1/$_2$ to 2^1/$_2$ years	3.77	451	1.02	1.14
2^1/$_2$ to 3^1/$_2$ years	13.42	544	1.57	1.07
3^1/$_2$ to 4^1/$_2$ years	27.75	537	2.20	1.14
All children	15.60	1532	1.12	1.21
Any treated caries				
1^1/$_2$ to 2^1/$_2$ years	0.22	451	0.24	1.08
2^1/$_2$ to 3^1/$_2$ years	0.92	544	0.37	0.91
3^1/$_2$ to 4^1/$_2$ years	7.08	537	1.09	0.98
All children	2.87	1532	0.41	0.95
Any trauma of incisors				
1^1/$_2$ to 2^1/$_2$ years	11.18	474	1.41	0.97
2^1/$_2$ to 3^1/$_2$ years	18.17	556	1.66	1.01
3^1/$_2$ to 4^1/$_2$ years	16.30	540	1.54	0.97
All children	15.44	1570	0.95	1.04
Any trauma to upper incisors				
1^1/$_2$ to 2^1/$_2$ years	10.53	474	1.31	0.93
2^1/$_2$ to 3^1/$_2$ years	17.45	556	1.65	1.02
3^1/$_2$ to 4^1/$_2$ years	15.37	540	1.50	0.96
All children	14.64	1570	0.90	1.01
Any buccal erosion				
1^1/$_2$ to 2^1/$_2$ years	7.14	462	1.98	1.65
2^1/$_2$ to 3^1/$_2$ years	9.91	545	1.83	1,43
3^1/$_2$ to 4^1/$_2$ years	13.79	515	2.24	1.48
All children	10.38	1522	1.68	2.15
Any buccal erosion into dentine or pulp				
1^1/$_2$ to 2^1/$_2$ years	1.30	462	0.57	1.09
2^1/$_2$ to 3^1/$_2$ years	2.20	545	0.65	1.04
3^1/$_2$ to 4^1/$_2$ years	2.91	515	0.70	0.94
All children	2.17	1522	0.40	1.06
Any palatal erosion				
1^1/$_2$ to 2^1/$_2$ years	9.21	445	2.06	1.50
2^1/$_2$ to 3^1/$_2$ years	18.39	533	2.23	1.33
3^1/$_2$ to 4^1/$_2$ years	29.15	518	2.44	1.22
All children	19.38	1496	1.76	1.72
Any palatal erosion into dentine or pulp				
1^1/$_2$ to 2^1/$_2$ years	3.15	445	0.82	0.99
2^1/$_2$ to 3^1/$_2$ years	6.19	533	1.10	1.05
3^1/$_2$ to 4^1/$_2$ years	12.93	518	1.62	1.10
All children	7.62	1496	0.81	1.17

Table 3 Proportion of children with different patterns of toothbrushing behaviour and the associated standard errors and design factors

Measure of dental behaviour	Percentage of children with characteristic % p	Sample size	Standard error of p	Design factor
Started toothbrushing aged less than one year				
1½ to 2½ years	53.62	497	2.12	0.95
2½ to 3½ years	47.90	598	2.40	1.17
3½ to 4½ years	46.57	559	2.21	1.04
All children	49.18	1654	1.46	1.18
Started toothbrushing aged 1 to 2 years				
1½ to 2½ years	41.53	497	2.31	1.04
2½ to 3½ years	41.85	598	2.17	1.07
3½ to 4½ years	37.55	559	2.15	1.05
All children	40.30	1654	1.42	1.17
Started toothbrushing aged 2 years and over				
1½ to 2½ years	1.01	497	0.41	0.91
2½ to 3½ years	8.74	598	1.16	1.01
3½ to 4½ years	15.34	559	1.72	1.12
All children	8.63	1654	0.76	1.09
Has not started toothbrushing				
1½ to 2½ years	3.83	497	1.04	1.21
2½ to 3½ years	1.51	598	0.44	0.89
3½ to 4½ years	0.54	559	0.24	0.75
All children	1.88	1654	0.37	1.09
Teeth brushed less than once a day				
1½ to 2½ years	13.88	497	1.85	1.19
2½ to 3½ years	12.42	598	1.44	1.07
3½ to 4½ years	10.02	559	1.14	0.90
All children	12.05	1654	0.94	1.17
Teeth brushed once a day				
1½ to 2½ years	38.03	497	2.27	1.04
2½ to 3½ years	32.05	598	1.58	0.83
3½ to 4½ years	30.41	559	2.01	1.03
All children	33.29	1654	1.28	1.11
Teeth brushed more than once a day				
1½ to 2½ years	48.09	497	2.21	0.98
2½ to 3½ years	55.54	598	1.92	0.94
3½ to 4½ years	59.57	559	2.41	1.16
All children	54.66	1654	1.41	1.15

Table 4 True standard errors and design factors for certain behavioural characteristics of the dental sample

Characteristic	Percentage of children with characteristic % p	Sample size	Standard error of p	Design factor
Used a bottle	87.42	1654	1.30	1.60
Used a dinky feeder	17.96	1654	1.43	1.51
Used a dummy	53.33	1654	1.40	1.14
Used a teething aid	91.17	1654	0.80	1.15
Received advice on some aspect of dental care	60.07	1654	1.53	1.27
Used fluoride supplements				
1½ to 2½ years	16.10	497	1.97	1.20
2½ to 3½ years	17.92	598	1.78	1.13
3½ to 4½ years	20.39	559	2.12	1.24
All children	18.21	1654	1.42	1.50
Reported to consume sugar confectionery on most days of the week or more frequently				
1½ to 2½ years	32.60	497	2.52	1.20
2½ to 3½ years	46.91	598	2.26	1.11
3½ to 4½ years	47.05	559	2.05	0.97
Reported to consume carbonated drinks on most days of the week or more frequently				
1½ to 2½ years	16.10	497	1.78	1.08
2½ to 3½ years	26.50	598	2.08	1.16
3½ to 4½ years	29.34	559	2.27	1.18

Table 5 Standard errors and design factors associated with different frequencies of having a drink in bed at night and the type of vessel used for night-time drink

Frequency of having a drink in bed at night and vessel used when drink in bed	Percentage of children with characteristic % p	Sample size	Standard error of p	Design factor
Frequency of having a drink in bed				
Every night				
$1^1/_2$ to $2^1/_2$ years	39.44	497	2.35	1.07
$2^1/_2$ to $3^1/_2$ years	31.94	598	2.05	1.07
$3^1/_2$ to $4^1/_2$ years	22.04	559	1.83	1.04
All children	30.85	1654	1.33	1.17
1 - 6 nights a week				
$1^1/_2$ to $2^1/_2$ years	7.04	497	1.03	0.90
$2^1/_2$ to $3^1/_2$ years	9.87	598	1.35	1.11
$3^1/_2$ to $4^1/_2$ years	13.26	559	1.45	1.01
All children	10.16	1654	0.69	0.93
Less than once a week				
$1^1/_2$ to $2^1/_2$ years	4.63	497	1.18	1.25
$2^1/_2$ to $3^1/_2$ years	6.35	598	1.07	1.07
$3^1/_2$ to $4^1/_2$ years	8.96	559	1.15	0.95
All children	6.72	1654	0.72	1.18
Never				
$1^1/_2$ to $2^1/_2$ years	48.89	497	2.38	1.06
$2^1/_2$ to $3^1/_2$ years	51.84	598	2.14	1.05
$3^1/_2$ to $4^1/_2$ years	55.73	559	2.50	1.19
All children	52.27	1654	1.71	1.39
Drinking vessel used in bed				
Bottle				
$1^1/_2$ to $2^1/_2$ years	32.66	497	2.32	1.09
$2^1/_2$ to $3^1/_2$ years	16.81	598	1.67	1.09
$3^1/_2$ to $4^1/_2$ years	6.08	559	0.99	0.98
Feeder beaker				
$1^1/_2$ to $2^1/_2$ years	12.98	497	1.28	0.84
$2^1/_2$ to $3^1/_2$ years	15.64	598	1.67	1.13
$3^1/_2$ to $4^1/_2$ years	9.48	559	1.43	1.15
Mug, cup or glass				
$1^1/_2$ to $2^1/_2$ years	3.44	497	0.80	0.97
$2^1/_2$ to $3^1/_2$ years	14.31	598	1.60	1.12
$3^1/_2$ to $4^1/_2$ years	28.09	559	1.80	0.95

Table 6 Standard errors and design factors associated with having different drinks in bed at night

Drinks in bed at night	Percentage of children	Sample size	Standard error of p	Design factor
Milk				
$1^1/_2$ to $2^1/_2$ years	23.98	497	1.58	0.82
$2^1/_2$ to $3^1/_2$ years	16.30	598	1.39	0.91
$3^1/_2$ to $4^1/_2$ years	9.17	559	1.37	1.12
All children	16.17	1654	0.88	0.97
Water				
$1^1/_2$ to $2^1/_2$ years	7.17	497	1.20	1.02
$2^1/_2$ to $3^1/_2$ years	9.85	598	1.26	1.02
$3^1/_2$ to $4^1/_2$ years	13.67	559	1.51	1.04
All children	10.35	1654	0.82	1.08
Drink containing NME sugars				
$1^1/_2$ to $2^1/_2$ years	11.89	497	1.71	1.16
$2^1/_2$ to $3^1/_2$ years	11.71	598	1.11	0.84
$3^1/_2$ to $4^1/_2$ years	12.23	559	1.69	1.22
All children	11.94	1654	0.88	1.10
Other drink, not containing NME sugars				
$1^1/_2$ to $2^1/_2$ years	7.17	497	1.34	1.14
$2^1/_2$ to $3^1/_2$ years	9.51	598	1.29	1.07
$3^1/_2$ to $4^1/_2$ years	8.81	559	1.13	0.94
All children	8.57	1654	0.72	1.04

Table 7 Average daily intake of selected foods containing sugars and certain nutrients and the associated standard errors and design factors

Weighed intake data

Intake of foods containing sugars and selected nutrients	Mean daily intake (g)	Sample size	Standard error of mean	Design factor
Foods containg sugars:				
Sugar confectionery (g)				
1½ to 2½ years	5.91	465	0.61	1.17
2½ to 3½ years	10.03	566	0.68	1.13
3½ to 4½ years	12.24	537	0.73	1.03
Chocolate confectionery (g)				
1½ to 2½ years	8.38	465	0.51	1.05
2½ to 3½ years	11.69	566	0.53	0.99
3½ to 4½ years	11.73	537	0.57	1.01
Soft drinks (g) *				
1½ to 2½ years	229.11	465	14.07	1.09
2½ to 3½ years	268.34	566	12.29	1.06
3½ to 4½ years	278.47	537	12.15	1.07
Fruit juice (g)				
1½ to 2½ years	39.01	465	3.95	0.99
2½ to 3½ years	37.77	566	4.03	1.16
3½ to 4½ years	35.46	537	3.52	1.07
Various foods containing sugars (g)†				
1½ to 2½ years	353.41	465	15.01	1.11
2½ to 3½ years	406.84	566	12.99	1.06
3½ to 4½ years	423.91	537	14.00	1.19
Selected nutrients§:				
Total sugars (g)				
1½ to 2½ years	80.60	465	1.39	1.05
2½ to 3½ years	88.46	566	1.17	0.99
3½ to 4½ years	99.31	537	1.55	1.19
Non-milk extrinsic sugars (g)				
1½ to 2½ years	48.64	465	1.31	1.04
2½ to 3½ years	59.27	566	1.11	0.99
3½ to 4½ years	64.53	537	1.49	1.24
Intrinsic and milk sugars and starch (g)				
1½ to 2½ years	89.74	465	1.04	0.97
2½ to 3½ years	97.19	566	0.99	0.98
3½ to 4½ years	105.23	537	1.18	1.05
Carbohydrate (g)				
1½ to 2½ years	138.61	465	1.68	1.00
2½ to 3½ years	156.54	566	1.45	0.95
3½ to 4½ years	169.82	537	1.81	1.13

* Includes fruit squashes with sugar and carbonated drinks, including low-calorie carbonated drinks.

† Includes intakes from the following food groups: biscuits; buns; cakes; pastries; fruit pies; milk, sponge and other puddings; ice cream; yogurt; fruit in syrup; sugar; preserves; sugar confectionery; chocolate confectionery; fruit juice; other soft drinks.

§ Nutrient variables measuring actual intakes of sugars/nutrients within all foods, including intakes from dietary supplements.

Table 8 Average daily frequency of consumption of selected foods containing sugars and the associated standard errors and design factors

Weighed intake data

Foods containing sugars	Mean daily frequency of consumption	Sample size	Standard error of mean	Design factor
Sugar confectionery				
1$\frac{1}{2}$ to 2$\frac{1}{2}$ years	0.24	465	0.02	1.24
2$\frac{1}{2}$ to 3$\frac{1}{2}$ years	0.40	566	0.03	1.24
3$\frac{1}{2}$ to 4$\frac{1}{2}$ years	0.45	537	0.02	0.99
Chocolate confectionery				
1$\frac{1}{2}$ to 2$\frac{1}{2}$ years	0.41	465	0.02	1.10
2$\frac{1}{2}$ to 3$\frac{1}{2}$ years	0.48	566	0.02	1.03
3$\frac{1}{2}$ to 4$\frac{1}{2}$ years	0.45	537	0.02	1.07
Soft drinks*				
1$\frac{1}{2}$ to 2$\frac{1}{2}$ years	1.51	465	0.09	1.22
2$\frac{1}{2}$ to 3$\frac{1}{2}$ years	1.71	566	0.07	1.05
3$\frac{1}{2}$ to 4$\frac{1}{2}$ years	1.63	537	0.07	1.07
Fruit juice				
1$\frac{1}{2}$ to 2$\frac{1}{2}$ years	0.41	465	0.04	0.96
2$\frac{1}{2}$ to 3$\frac{1}{2}$ years	0.36	566	0.04	1.16
3$\frac{1}{2}$ to 4$\frac{1}{2}$ years	0.31	537	0.03	1.05
Various foods containing sugars†				
1$\frac{1}{2}$ to 2$\frac{1}{2}$ years	5.02	465	0.13	1.09
2$\frac{1}{2}$ to 3$\frac{1}{2}$ years	5.56	566	0.11	1.02
3$\frac{1}{2}$ to 4$\frac{1}{2}$ years	5.56	537	0.10	1.06

* Includes fruit squashes with sugar and carbonated drinks, including low-calorie carbonated drinks.
† Includes intakes from the following food groups: biscuits; buns; cakes; pastries; fruit pies; milk, sponge and other puddings; ice cream; yogurt; fruit in syrup; sugar; preserves; sugar confectionery; chocolate confectionery; fruit juice; other soft drinks.

References and notes

[1] Gregory J R Collins D L Davies P S W Hughes J M Clarke P C. National Diet and Nutrition Survey: children aged 1$\frac{1}{2}$ to 4$\frac{1}{2}$ years. Volume 1: *Report of the diet and nutrition survey* HMSO (1995)

[2] Epsilon was developed by Social Survey Division for samples drawn using multi-stage sample designs. For further details of the method of calculation see Butcher B and Elliott D *A sampling errors manual*. OPCS; NM13, (1987).

[3] Where the actual difference between p_1 and p_2 > value obtained from calculation, the difference is significant at the given level.

[4] Where the actual difference between mean$_1$ and mean$_2$ > value obtained from calculation, the difference is significant at the given level.

Appendix G Glossary of abbreviations, terms and survey definitions

Active decay (dental) Untreated dental *caries* including decay into the enamel, dentine and dental pulp (see Appendix A for classification criteria).

Benefits (receiving) Receipt of Income Support or Family Credit by the child's mother or her husband/partner.

Buccal (surface) Front surface of an incisor (visible when smiling).

Canine Tooth located between the incisors and deciduous molars (2 in each jaw).

Caries (dental) Disease of the teeth - tooth decay.

Cariogenic (foods) Foods thought to be particularly likely to contribute to development of *caries*.

Central incisors see *Incisors*.

CSE Certificate of Secondary Education.

Cum % Cumulative percentage (of a distribution).

Decay experience A tooth with decay experience can have *active decay* or be *filled* or *missing* due to decay.

Deciduous (dentition) The first set of teeth to erupt into the mouth, which are shed between the ages of about 6 and 11 years and replaced with the permanent teeth (also known as primary dentition).

Dental caries see *caries*.

Dentine Calcified tissue which forms the major part of a tooth (found between the *enamel* and *dental pulp*).

DH The Department of Health.

Diary sample Children for whom a four-day dietary record, covering two weekdays and both weekend days, was obtained.

Economically inactive Those neither working nor *unemployed;* includes students, the retired, individuals who were looking after the home or family and those permanently unable to work due to ill health or disability.

Economic status Whether at the time of interview the individual was *working, unemployed,* or *economically inactive.*

Enamel (dental) The hard outer layer of a tooth.

Erosion (dental) Progressive loss of dental hard tissue by a chemical process that does not involve bacteria.

Extractions/ extracted teeth Extracted teeth are those which have been removed by a dentist see *Missing* teeth (see also Appendix A).

Extrinsic sugars Any sugar which is not contained within the cell walls of a food. Examples are the sugars in honey, table sugar and lactose in milk and milk products (see also notes to Chapter 5).

Family unit and family type *Family units* exist within a *household* and describe the relationship of household members to each other. A family unit can consist of:
(a) a married or cohabiting couple on their own, or
(b) a married or cohabiting couple/ lone parent and their never married children; provided these children have no children of their own, or
(c) one person on their own.
All family units in this survey included never married children. *Family type* distinguishes between children living in family units with two parents, and those living in family units with a lone parent.

Filled (teeth) Teeth with a permanent restoration (filling) of any material, and no *active decay.*

GCE General Certificate of Education.

GHS The General Household Survey; a continuous, multi-purpose household survey, carried out by the Social Survey Division of OPCS on behalf of a number of government departments.

Head of household The head of household is defined as follows:
(a) in a household containing only a husband, wife and children under age 16 years (and boarders), the **husband** is always the head of household.
(b) in a cohabiting household the **male partner** is always the head of household.
(c) when the household comprises other relatives and/or unrelated persons the **owner, or the person legally responsible** for the accommodation, is always the head of the household.

In cases where more than one person has equal claim, the following rules apply:
(i) where they are of the same sex, the oldest is always the head of household
(ii) where they are of different sex the male is always the head of household.

Household The standard definition used in most surveys carried out by OPCS Social Survey Division, and comparable with the 1991 Census definition of a household was used in this survey. A household is defined as a single person or group of people who have the accommodation as their only or main residence and who either share one main meal a day or share the living accommodation. (See E McCrossan *A Handbook for interviewers.* HMSO:1985.)

Highest educational qualification Based on the highest educational qualification obtained by the child's mother, grouped as follows:

GCE 'A' level or above
Degree (or degree level qualification)
Teaching qualification

128

| Highest educational qualification - *continued* | HNC/HND, BEC/TEC Higher, BTEC City and Guilds Full Technological Certificate
Nursing qualifications (SRN, SCM, RGN, RM, RHV, Midwife)
GCE 'A' level/SCE higher
ONC/OND/BEC/TEC <u>not</u> higher |

'Other qualifications'

GCE 'O' level passes (Grades A-C if after 1975)
GCSE (Grades A-C)
CSE (Grade 1)
SCE Ordinary (Bands A-C)
Standard Grade (Levels 1-3)
SLC Lower
SUPE Lower or Ordinary
School Certificate or Matriculation
City and Guilds Craft/Ordinary Level
CSE Grades 2-5, and ungraded
GCE 'O' Level (Grades D and E if after 1975)
GCSE (Grades D-G)
SCE Ordinary (Bands D and E)
Standard Grade (Levels 4 and 5)
Clerical or commercial qualifications
Apprenticeship
Other qualifications

None
No educational qualifications

The qualification levels do not in all cases correspond to those used in statistics published by the Department for Education.

Incisors	Front four teeth in each jaw. The front two teeth in each jaw are known as central incisors and the other incisors are referred to as lateral incisors.
Intrinsic sugars	Any sugar which is contained within the cell wall of a food (see also notes to Chapter 5).
Lateral incisors	see *Incisors*.
MAFF	The Ministry of Agriculture, Fisheries and Food.
Manual social class	Children living in households where the head of household was in an occupation ascribed to *Social Classes III manual, IV or V*.
Median	see *Quantiles*.
Missing (teeth)	Teeth which had erupted, but were not present in the mouth at the time of examination were assumed to have been *extracted* as a result of decay, unless they were known to have been lost through *trauma*.
Molar	Grinding tooth situated at the back of the mouth. In the *deciduous* dentition there are four molars in each jaw.
NDNS	The National Diet and Nutrition Survey.
NHS	National Health Service.
Non-manual social classes	Children living in households where the head of household was in an occupation ascribed to *Social Classes I, II or III non-manual*.
Non-milk extrinsic (NME) sugars	*Extrinsic sugars*, except lactose in milk and milk products (see also notes to Chapter 5).
OPCS	The Office of Population Censuses and Surveys.

PAF	Postcode Address File; the sampling frame for the survey.
Palatal (surface)	Back (throat facing) surface of an *incisor*.
Percentiles	see *Quantiles*.
PSU	Primary Sampling Unit; for this survey, postcode sectors.
Pulp (dental)	Soft vascular tissue which fills the pulp chamber and the root canals of a tooth. It consists of connective tissue, blood vessels and nerves (the inner most part of the tooth).
Quantiles	The quantiles of a distribution divide it into equal parts. The *median* of a distribution divides it into two equal parts, such that half the cases in the distribution fall, or have a value, above the median, and the other half fall, or have a value below the median. *Percentiles* divide the distribution into 100 equal parts; at the tenth percentile there will be one value; 90% of cases will fall, or have a value above the 10th percentile and 10% of cases will fall, or have a value below the 10th percentile (see also note in Chapter 6).

| Region | Based on the Standard regions and grouped as follows: |

Scotland

Northern
North
Yorkshire and Humberside
North West

Central, South West and Wales
East Midlands
West Midlands
East Anglia
South West
Wales

London and South East
London
South East

The regions of England are as constituted after local government reorganisation on 1 April 1974. The regions as defined in terms of counties are listed at the back of this Appendix; a map of Great Britain showing the regions is given as Figure G1.

Responding sample	Informants who co-operated with any part of the survey.
se	Standard error of estimate; see *Appendix F* for method of calculation.
Social Class	Based on the Registrar General's *Standard Occupational Classification*, Volume 3 HMSO (1991). Social class was ascribed on the basis of the occupation of the head of household. The classification used in the tables is as follows:

Descriptive definition Social class

Non-manual	
Professional and intermediate	I and II
Skilled occupations, non manual	III non-manual

Manual	
Skilled occupations, manual	III manual
Partly-skilled and unskilled occupations	IV and V

Social class - *continued*

Social class was not determined for households where the head had never worked, was a full-time student, was in the Armed Forces or whose occupation was inadequately described. If the head of household was male, social class was determined on the basis of their present, main occupation or, if they were currently unemployed, on the basis of the last occupation and if they were waiting to take up a new job, on the basis of that new occupation. If the head of household was female, social class was determined on the basis of what the informant regarded as her 'main' life occupation.

State of the teeth (examination)

Component of the dental examination to identify presence of dental *caries*: coded as *active decay*, *filled teeth* or teeth *missing* due to decay.

Trauma (dental)

Accidental damage to a tooth ranging from discolouration or fractured enamel to loss of the tooth.

Unemployed

Those actively seeking work, those intending to look for work but prevented by sickness (28 days or fewer) and those waiting to take up a job already obtained.

Unerupted (tooth)

A tooth was unerupted if it had not erupted into the mouth, that is no part of the tooth was visible.

Working

In paid work, as an employee or self employed, at any time in the 7 days prior to the interview or not working in the 7 days prior to interview but with a job to return to, including, for women, being on maternity leave.

Figure G1 Standard Regions of England, Scotland and Wales and aggregated regions for analysis

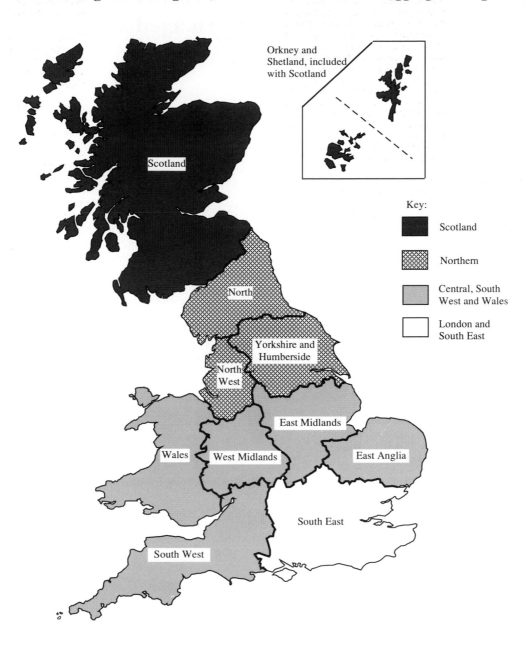

North
Tyne and Wear Metropolitan County
Cleveland
Cumbria
Durham
Northumberland

Yorkshire and Humberside
South Yorkshire Metropolitan County
West Yorkshire Metropolitan County
Humberside
North Yorkshire

East Midlands
Derbyshire
Leicestershire
Lincolnshire
Northamptonshire
Nottinghamshire

East Anglia
Cambridgeshire
Norfolk
Suffolk

South East

Greater London
Bedfordshire
Berkshire
Buckinghamshire
East Sussex
Essex
Hampshire
Hertfordshire
Isle of Wight
Kent
Oxfordshire
Surrey
West Sussex

South West
Avon
Cornwall and Isles of Scilly
Devon
Dorset
Gloucestershire
Somerset
Wiltshire

West Midlands
West Midlands Metropolitan County
Hereford and Worcester
Shropshire
Staffordshire
Warwickshire

North West
Greater Manchester Metropolitan County
Merseyside Metropolitan County
Cheshire
Lancashire

131

Appendix H Summary taken from the report of National Diet and Nutrition Survey: children aged $1^1/_2$ to $4^1/_2$ years

Vol 1: Report of Diet and Nutrition Survey

Summary

Introduction

This Report presents the findings of a survey of the diet and nutrition of British children aged 1½ to 4½ years carried out between July 1992 and June 1993. The survey forms part of the National Diet and Nutrition Survey programme which was set up jointly by the Ministry of Agriculture, Fisheries and Food and the Department of Health in 1992 following the successful Dietary and Nutritional Survey of British Adults[1]. This cross-sectional study of children aged 1½ to 4½ years is part of a planned programme of surveys covering representative samples of defined age groups of the population. Other groups to follow will be older adults aged 65 years or over and school children aged 5 to 15 years, before returning to adults aged 16 to 64 years. Preschool children were chosen as the first of the new groups because no nationally representative survey had been undertaken since the Government survey by the Health Departments in 1967/8[2].

The children in the survey

A nationally representative sample of 2101 children aged 1½ to 4½ years was identified from a postal sift of addresses selected from the Postcode Address File. Only children living in private households were eligible to be included and only one child per household was selected. The interview, which was the first stage of the full survey protocol, was completed for 1859 children (88% of the identified sample). These 1859 children are referred to as the interview sample. The numbers of children in the interview sample were 648 aged 1½ to 2½ years, 668 aged 2½ to 3½ years and 543 aged 3½ to 4½ years. The survey fieldwork covered 12 months to take account of possible seasonal variation in eating habits.

(Chapters 1 and 3 and Appendix C).

The interview sample of children was found to be representative of the population in terms of social and demographic characteristics as assessed by reference to the 1992 General Household Survey[3] and mid year population estimates[4]. *(Chapter 3).*

The survey design included an interview, generally with the child's mother, to provide information about socio-demographic circumstances of the child's household, medication and eating and drinking habits; a weighed dietary record of all food and drink consumed over four consecutive days (including a Saturday and Sunday); a record of bowel movements for the same four days; physical measurements of the child (weight, standing height, mid upper-arm and head circumferences, and supine length for children under 2 years of age); a request for a sample of blood; and a dental examination.

Records of weighed dietary intake were obtained for 1675 children, that is 90% of those completing the interview and 80% of those identified by the sift. Physical measurements were obtained for over 90% of the interview sample. Consent to the request for a blood sample was given for 1157 children (63% of the interview sample) and blood was obtained from 1003 children (54%). The final element in the survey was an assessment of dental health by questionnaire and examination. An examination and/or dental interview was achieved for 1658 children, that is 89% of the children for whom a dietary interview had been obtained. This final element in the survey took place at the end of each of the four 3-month dietary survey fieldwork periods. A full Report of this dental survey is published separately as Volume 2[5]. A summary of the dental survey is at Appendix Q.

The foods and drinks consumed

The proportion of children consuming the various foods was based on the numbers of consumers during the four-day period of recording, which would not necessarily be the same as the proportion of these same children consuming these foods over any longer period. An explanation of the method used to re-weight the food intake data and estimate the average daily intake of nutrients is provided in Appendix J. The following foods and drinks were consumed by more than 70% of the children during the four-day recording period; biscuits; white bread; non-diet soft drinks; whole milk; savoury snacks (includes both potato crisps and cereal-based snacks); boiled, mashed or jacket potatoes; chocolate confectionery and chips. Coated or fried white fish had been eaten by 38%, but white fish cooked by methods other than frying by only 10%, and oily fish by 16% of children. Fifty nine percent of the children had eaten some cheese but the amounts were small, 40% of children had eaten yogurt and 46% eggs. Of fats and oils, polyunsaturated margarine was consumed by the largest proportion of children (36%) and butter by 30%. Sausages, chicken and turkey, and beef and beef dishes were eaten by about half of the children. Peas and carrots were the only cooked vegetables, excluding potatoes, to be eaten by more than half the children (carrots, 54% and peas 53%). Of any vegetable, baked beans were consumed in the greatest quantities and were eaten by 49% of all children in the survey. Leafy green vegetables were eaten by only 39% and in fairly small quantities. Raw vegetables and salad were eaten by less than 24% of children during the four-day period. The most popular fruits were apples and pears, then bananas. Chocolate confectionery was more commonly eaten than sugar confectionery, by 74% and 58% of children respectively.

(Chapter 4)

In the interview mothers reported that whole milk was given as a drink to 68% of children while 19% usually had semi-skimmed and 1% skimmed milk to drink. In all, 8% of the children were reported as having no milk to drink although some of these had it mixed with food, for example, on cereals and in milk puddings. Soft drinks were consumed by the majority of children. Half of those drinking non-diet soft drinks were estimated to be consuming about 1.5 litres a week and half of those who drank diet soft drinks were consuming about 1 litre per week. Fruit juice and tea were each consumed by about one third of children but in smaller quantities.

(Chapter 4)

Twenty one percent of children were reported in the interview to be taking dietary supplements and information from the dietary records showed that 19% of the children had taken dietary supplements during the four days (11% as tablets, 3% as syrups and 5% as drops). Children who were reported as taking dietary supplements generally had higher intakes of vitamins from food than children who did not take supplements.

(Chapter 8)

When the successive age groups were compared, trends in eating patterns with age were identified. More of the youngest children ate bananas, commercial infant and toddlers' foods, fish which was neither coated or fried, yogurt and whole milk, while more of the older children ate white bread, buns, cakes and pastries, ice cream, sugar confectionery, meat products, chips and savoury snacks. The quantity of food consumed generally increased with age including the amounts of sugar and chocolate confectionery. However the mean consumption of whole milk decreased by almost one third from the youngest to the oldest age groups. There were small differences in the amounts of foods consumed by girls and by boys in the older age group. *(Chapter 4)*

Energy consumption

The mean daily energy intakes for children aged 1½ to 2½ years were 4393kJ (1045kcal), for those aged 2½ to 3½ years 4882kJ (1160kcal), and for the oldest group of girls intake was 4976kJ (1183kcal) compared with the oldest group of boys intake of 5356kJ (1273kcal).

(Chapter 5)

For each age/sex group the mean energy intakes were below the Estimated Average Requirements (EARs)[6]. It was considered unlikely that these recorded low levels of energy intakes were due to poor dietary recording methodology following the validation of the method using a doubly-labelled water technique in the feasibility study[7]. Values for EAR for energy for infants set in 1979[8] were revised and lowered in 1991[6]. EAR values for older pre-school children were also slightly revised in 1991, but may still be set too high. The mean energy intakes of subjects in this study probably do not reflect inadequate amounts for the maintenance of health and growth. When compared with the children examined in the Government survey of 1967/8[2], children of the same age in 1992/3 were on average significantly taller *(Fig 11.2)*.

At all ages cereals and cereal products made the largest contribution to energy intake (overall 30%), and this was closely followed by milk and milk products (overall 20%), then vegetables, potatoes and savoury snacks (overall 12%) *(Table 5.7b and Fig 5.6)*. The proportion of energy from milk and milk products reduced from 26% for the youngest age group to 16% for the oldest children whereas the proportion of energy from cereals and cereal products increased from 27% for the youngest group to 32% for the oldest group of children *(Fig 5.6)*. On average children in the sample derived about one fifth of their mean energy intake from foods eaten away from home. The amount of energy derived from each of the macronutrients, protein, carbohydrate and fat for each of the three age groups and for boys and girls is shown in the table below and in *Figure 6.3*.

Macronutrient contribution to food energy intake by age and sex of child

| | Age and sex of child | | | | | | |
| | All aged 1½–2½ years | All aged 2½–3½ years | All aged 3½–4½ years | | All boys | All girls | All |
			Boys	Girls			
Average daily intake:							
Total food energy (kcal)	1045	1160	1273	1181	1172	1108	1141
Total food energy (kJ)	4393	4882	5356	4976	4930	4663	4798
Protein (g)	35.4	36.8	39.4	37.7	37.4	36.2	36.8
Carbohydrate (g)	139	159	177	162	160	150	155
Total fat (g)	42.5	46.3	50.1	47.2	46.7	44.6	45.7
Percentage food energy from:							
Protein (%)	13.6	12.7	12.4	12.7	12.8	13.1	13.0
Carbohydrate (%)	49.9	51.5	52.3	51.7	51.4	50.8	51.1
Fat (%)	36.4	35.8	35.3	35.5	35.7	36.1	35.9

The nutrients: protein

The mean protein intake for all children was 36.8g which contributed about 13% of the total food energy. Children aged 1½ to 2½ years obtained a slightly higher proportion of their energy from protein than older children. Mean intakes of protein for each group defined by age and sex, in all cases, considerably exceeded the Reference Nutrient Intake (RNI)[6]. Milk and milk products (overall 33%), then cereals and cereal products (overall 23%) and meat and meat products (overall 22%) all made major contributions to protein intake.

(Chapter 6)

The nutrients: carbohydrates including non-starch polysaccharides (dietary fibre)

The mean daily carbohydrate intake (excluding non-starch polysaccharides) for all children was 155g which contributed about 51% of the total food energy. The average daily intake of total sugars for all children was 87g which contributed 29% of the total food energy and that of starch was 68g which contributed 22% of total food energy. Total sugars have been further subdivided into non-milk extrinsic sugars and intrinsic and milk sugars. Non-milk extrinsic sugars provided on average about 19% of total food energy. The main dietary sources of non-milk extrinsic sugars were soft drinks, which contributed a third of the total, followed by confectionery which contributed about one fifth. Other major contributors were biscuits (7%) and fruit juices (6%).

(Chapter 6)

Of the starch in the diets of these children two thirds was obtained from cereals and cereal products and about a quarter was obtained from vegetables, potatoes and savoury snacks. The intakes of total starch increased with age and also provided an increasing proportion of energy intake with increasing age of the child. When intrinsic and milk sugars were added to starch they contributed overall 32% of the total food energy.

(Chapter 6)

The average daily intake of non-starch polysaccharides (NSP) was 6.1g. However intakes increased with age with the youngest children having an average daily intake of 5.5g and the oldest boys 6.8g (oldest girls 6.4g) *(Table 6.20)*. The main dietary sources of NSP were vegetables (excluding potatoes) (17%), potatoes including fried potatoes (13%), high fibre and whole grain breakfast cereals (12%) and fruit (11%) with a smaller contribution from bread (white 7% and wholemeal 6%) *(Table 6.21b)*. There was a positive correlation between increasing levels of NSP intake and numbers of bowel movements daily.

(Chapter 6)

Dietary fats and blood lipids

The average daily total fat intake for all children was 45.7g which contributed 35.9% of total food energy. Saturated fatty acids contributed an average of 16.2% of total food energy. The proportion of energy from total fat and saturated fatty acids tended to decline with increasing age, from 36.4% and 16.9% respectively for the youngest age group to 35.3% from total fat and 15.4% from saturated fatty acids for boys in the oldest age group and 35.5% from total fat and 15.5% from saturated fatty acids for girls in the oldest age group. The main food sources of total fat were milk and milk products (35% at 1½ to 2½ years; 26% at 2½ to 3½ years and 22% for both boys and girls in the oldest age group). Cereals and cereal products contributed one fifth of the total fat and meat and meat products contributed one sixth overall. Milk, meat, savoury snacks and biscuits were major contributors of saturated fatty acids in the diet.

(Chapter 7)

Trans fatty acids provided about 1.7% of total food energy from an average daily intake of between 2.0 to 2.4g. Most *trans* fatty acids were derived from cows' milk (21%), fat spreads (14%), biscuits (13%), buns, cakes and pastries (8%) *(Table 7.18a and b)*.

Cis-monounsaturated fatty acids provided about 11% of food energy. These were mainly derived from meat and meat products (20%), cows' milk (17%), savoury snacks (8%), fat spreads (8%), biscuits (6%) and fried potatoes (6%). The average intake of *cis* polyunsaturated fatty acids of the n-3 series contributed less than 1% of food energy which came in small amounts from fried potatoes, fish, meat, milk and cereal products. *Cis* n-6 polyunsaturated fatty acids contributed about 4% of total food energy, the main sources in the children's diets being polyunsaturated fat spreads, fried potatoes, meat and meat products, cereals and cereal products and milk.

Blood lipid results are reported for plasma total cholesterol, high density lipoprotein (HDL) cholesterol and for plasma triglycerides. The blood was not taken with the child fasting and therefore the values relating to triglyceride levels must be interpreted with caution. Plasma levels of both total and HDL cholesterol generally correlated positively (blood levels increasing as dietary intakes increased) with intakes of total fat, saturated, *trans* and *cis* monounsaturated fatty acids and with dietary cholesterol. However these relationships were generally weak, particularly with respect to levels of plasma total cholesterol. There was no consistent association between plasma total cholesterol and HDL cholesterol levels and intakes of *cis* n-3 and *cis* n-6 polyunsaturated fatty acids. *(Table 10.43)*.

(Chapter 10)

The nutrients: vitamins

Vitamin A intakes were derived from an assessment of daily retinol intakes with a contribution from carotenoid precursors of vitamin A combined as 'retinol equivalent'. The mean daily intake from food and dietary supplements for the whole group of children was 578µg. The skewed distribution of intakes of vitamin A (retinol equivalents) resulted in the median intake being lower than the mean intake, 428µg daily. About half of the children had average daily intakes of vitamin A which fell below the RNI value of 400µg. Eight percent of children aged under 4 years and 7% of children aged 4 years and over had intakes of vitamin A below the lower reference nutrient intake (LRNI) level. The food sources of vitamin A were mainly milk and vegetables. Overall liver provided about one sixth of total intake although only 4% of children had eaten it in the four-day recording period. Dietary supplements containing vitamin A contributed substantial amounts but they tended to be taken by children who were already towards the upper end of the range of intake levels. *(Chapter 8)*

Blood was analysed for retinol and several carotenoids. There were no clear associations between plasma retinol levels and dietary intakes of pre-formed retinol and total carotene. *(Chapter 10)*

On average the mean daily intakes for thiamin, ribo-flavin, niacin, vitamin B_6, vitamin B_{12} and folate were well above the RNI values. The average daily intakes for all children from both food sources and dietary supplements (that is, all sources) were for thiamin 0.8mg, for riboflavin 1.2mg, for niacin 16.3mg, for vitamin B_6 1.2mg, for vitamin B_{12} 2.8µg and for folate 132µg. None of the children aged under 4 years had intakes below the LRNI for niacin and vitamin B_{12} and only 1% or less had intakes below the LRNI for thiamin, riboflavin, vitamin B_6 and folate. Similarly none of the children aged 4 years and over had intakes below the LRNI for niacin and vitamin B_{12} and only 1% had intakes below the LRNI for thiamin, riboflavin and folate and 5% below that for vitamin B_6. The mean intakes of riboflavin per kilogram body weight declined from 0.1mg/kg to 0.07mg/kg with increasing age and this can be accounted for by the declining consumption of milk with increasing age. The range of intakes of vitamin C was wide and the distribution of intakes was skewed, with some children having intakes many times the RNI value. The mean daily intake from all sources was 51.8mg which was well above the RNI for vitamin C (30mg). Dietary supplements contributed 7% but none of the children in the bottom 2.5 percentile of intake took vitamin C supplements during the four days. Only 1% of all children had intake levels below the LRNI. *(Chapter 8)*

Results for blood analyses of the erythrocyte glutathione reductase activation coefficient (EGRAC), a measure of riboflavin status, and of vitamin B_{12}, red blood cell folate, plasma folate and vitamin C are reported. The data from this survey reflect, for the first time, levels of these analytes for the national population of children aged 1½ to 4½ years in Great Britain and thus provide population standards. The mean values for the blood samples provided by the children were for the EGRAC 1.24, for vitamin B_{12} 636pmol/l, for red cell folate 914nmol/l, and for plasma folate 21.1nmol/l *(Tables 10.17 to 10.21)*. Overall the mean level of plasma vitamin C was 67.6µmol/l, with a wide range between the lower and upper 2.5 percentiles (8.8µmol/l to 124.5 mol/l) *(Table 10.22 and Fig 10.4)*. There was almost no variation in plasma vitamin C by age but boys had significantly lower levels than girls. Dietary intakes of riboflavin for each age/sex cohort were significantly negatively correlated with the EGRAC. Red cell folate correlated positively with dietary intakes of folate and plasma levels of vitamin C with dietary intakes of vitamin C. *(Chapter 10)*

Average daily intakes of vitamin D from foods were low, 1.2µg in both the youngest and middle age groups and very slightly higher in the 3½ to 4½ years group (boys 1.4µg, girls 1.3µg). Dietary supplements resulted in an increase in total intakes to 1.8µg for both the youngest and middle groups and 2.0µg for the boys, 1.9µg for the girls in the 3½ to 4½ years group. The RNI at age 1 to 3 years is 7µg, a level met by only 5% of children aged under 4 years. No DRVs are set for vitamin D for children aged 4 years or over because most of the body's requirement for vitamin D in this age group can be synthesised by the skin if they are sufficiently exposed to sunlight. Children in the youngest age group, 1½ to 2½ years, were obtaining about one sixth of their mean daily intake of vitamin D from milk products, mainly infant formula, whereas boys in the oldest age group were obtaining only 5% and girls 2% from this food source. The other main food sources for all the children were breakfast cereals and fat spreads, many of which are fortified with vitamin D. *(Chapter 8)*

Blood levels of plasma 25-hydroxyvitamin D were determined and a mean value of 68.1nmol/l *(Table 10.34 and Fig 10.6)* was reported. There was no apparent association between the mean values and either the age or the sex of the child. However plasma vitamin D levels varied by season, with mean levels being highest in July to September and lowest in January to March *(Figure 10.7)*. In addition plasma levels correlated significantly with dietary intakes of vitamin D, plasma levels rising with increasing intakes. *(Chapter 10)*

The mean daily intake of vitamin E was 4.4mg for all children and there was a small increase with age from 3.9mg for the youngest age group to 5.1mg for boys and 4.6mg for girls in the oldest age group. Dietary supplements contributed only 2% to the intake of this vitamin. *(Chapter 8)*

Plasma α-and γ-tocopherols concentrations were measured. The mean plasma α-tocopherol level was 18.8µmol/l and the mean γ-tocopherol level was 1.6µmol/l. Levels of both tended to increase with age. Overall plasma α-tocopherol levels were positively correlated with total intakes of vitamin E. *(Chapter 10)*

The nutrients: minerals

Iron was the only mineral to which dietary supplements made a substantive contribution. Iron in the children's diet was assessed as haem iron (mainly found in meat) and non-haem iron. The average daily intake of total iron from food was 5.4mg, of which haem iron contributed only 4%. Dietary supplements increased the total iron intake by only 2% to 5.5mg daily. The average daily intakes were well below the RNI for iron, with 84% of those under 4 years of age and 57% of those aged 4 years and over having intakes below the RNI. Sixteen percent of those under 4 years of age had intakes from all sources below the LRNI which increased to 24% in those aged 1½ to 2½ years. The LRNI value for children aged 4 years and over is lower than for younger children and only 4% had intakes below the LRNI. The main food sources of iron were cereal products, many of which are fortified, vegetables, potatoes and savoury snacks and meat and meat products. *(Chapter 9)*

The mean haemoglobin concentration in samples from the children as a whole group was 12.2g/dl. Average values were lowest for the youngest group at 12.0g/dl and highest for boys aged 3½ to 4½ years at 12.4g/dl. Haemoglobin concentrations below 11.0g/dl were defined as an indication of anaemia[9]. One in eight in the youngest group were anaemic and one in 12 of all children were anaemic using this definition. Low ferritin levels also implied that a proportion of the children had poor iron status, with 20% of all children having ferritin levels below 10μg/l, and 5% having levels below 5μg/l. The ferritin levels matched the haemoglobin levels in that there was a higher proportion of children with low levels in the youngest age group. Other haematological measurements such as mean corpuscular volume (MCV), haematocrit, mean cell haemoglobin (MCH), and mean cell haemoglobin concentration (MCHC) as well as zinc protoporphyrin (ZPP) results all supported the haemoglobin and ferritin results to confirm that iron deficiency occurred commonly and that it was more prevalent in the youngest age group. Generally the correlations between haemoglobin, ferritin and ZPP and dietary intakes were weak. Only haemoglobin showed any significant correlation with intakes of total, haem and non-haem iron. *(Chapter 10)*

The mean daily intake for all children of calcium was 637mg, of phosphorus was 742mg and of magnesium was 136mg which for each of these minerals was well above the RNI values. The range of intakes of both calcium and phosphorus was large but for calcium only 1% of children under the age of 4 years and 2% of those aged 4 years and over had intakes below the LRNI. Likewise the proportions with intakes below the LRNI for magnesium were small, less than 1% of children aged under 4 years and 2% of those aged 4 years and over. The main source of calcium was milk and milk products which provided 64% of the mean intake. Average calcium intakes decreased markedly with age which reflects the decrease in milk consumption. Fortified cereals and cereal products are the second main source and the contribution from this source increased with age.

Sodium and chloride intakes (which do not include additions during cooking or at the table) were both, on average, more than twice the RNI values. For all children the estimated average daily intake of sodium was 1506mg and for chloride 2261mg. The mean daily intakes of potassium were 1476mg for children aged 1½ to 2½ years, 1513mg for those aged 2½ to 3½ years and 1501mg for girls in the oldest age group and 1573mg for boys in the oldest group. Average daily intakes were well in excess of the RNI values and only 1% or less of all children had intakes below the LRNI values.

Zinc intakes were generally below reference values. The average daily intake for children aged 1½ to 2½ years was 4.3mg and similar average intake was recorded for the middle age group. In the 3½ to 4½ years age group, the average intake for boys was 4.6mg and for girls 4.4mg. Seventy two percent of those aged under 4 years had intakes less than 5.0mg (the RNI value for this age

group) and 14% had mean intakes below 3.0mg (the LRNI value). A greater proportion of children aged 4 years and over had intakes below the RNI (89%) and LRNI (37%) values. The average intake of copper for children in the survey was 0.5mg. Thirty six percent of children aged under 4 years and 68% of those aged 4 years and over had intakes below the RNI. Average daily iodine intakes were above the RNI values, and only 3% of children aged under 4 years and 5% of those 4 years and over had intakes below the LRNIs. Intakes of manganese increased with age with a mean daily intake of 1.2mg for all children aged 1½ to 4½ years. *(Chapter 9)*

Blood samples were analysed for plasma zinc, which showed very little variation with either age or sex; the overall mean level was 13.0μmol/l. *(Chapter 10)*

Anthropometric measurements

The average weight of girls and boys aged 1½ to 2½ years was 11.9kg and 12.6kg respectively, of those 2½ to 3½ years group 14.3kg and 14.9kg and at age 3½ to 4½ years the average weights were 16.4kg and 16.6kg for girls and boys. The average standing heights were 86.9cm for boys and 85.3cm for girls in the youngest group, 95.6cm for boys and 94.7cm for girls in the middle age group and 102.1cm for boys and 101.3cm for girls in the 3½ to 4½ year age group. In addition, supine length was measured for children under 2 years of age. For boys supine length was on average 1.60cm greater than standing height; for girls the difference was 1.63cm. On average, the head circumferences of girls were smaller than those of boys. In the youngest age group the mean head circumference was 50.1cm for boys and 48.8cm for girls, and in the oldest age group the average measurements were 51.9cm for boys and 51.0cm for girls. Only in the youngest age group was there a significant difference in the mid upper-arm circumference between boys, 16.5cm and girls, 16.2cm. At 2½ to 3½ years arm circumferences were 17.0cm for both boys and girls and at 3½ to 4½ years arm circumferences were 17.5cm and 17.6cm respectively. When these measurements were compared with the results from the 1967/8 survey of children of a similar age, children today in the youngest age group were slightly lighter, boys aged 2½ to 4½ years were about the same average weight and girls aged 2½ to 4½ years were slightly heavier. There had been estimated increases in average heights between the two surveys of up to 3.5cm.

The body mass index (BMI) of children aged 3½ to 4½ years was the same for both sexes, 15.9. At younger ages boys had BMIs greater than girls. As was reported for the 1967/8 survey food energy intakes were correlated positively with BMI and arm circumference. *(Chapter 11)*

Unwell children

Twenty seven percent of the children were reported as being unwell at some time during the dietary recording period, and for 16% mothers reported that being unwell had affected their eating. For this latter group being unwell resulted in a mean energy intake about 13% lower than the mean intake for children who were well. For those for whom it had been reported that being unwell had not affected their eating habits mean energy intake was about 6% lower than that for children who were well *(Table 5.3a)*.

The children who were reported as being unwell during the dietary recording period had lower average intakes of protein, all carbohydrates, total fat and fatty acids, most vitamins and minerals than other children; this generally applied whether or not their eating was reported to have been affected by their illness. Most differences were associated with differences in energy intake between well and unwell children and not to the nutrient density of their diet.

Region

The nationally representative sample of children was subdivided into four regions for purposes of analyses based on where the child was living at the time of interview (see *Fig 3.1*).

There were differences in the proportions of children eating the various foods between the regions but patterns of eating behaviour associated with region were not always distinct. However, children in the Northern region were the most likely, and children in the London and the South East the least likely to be eating meat pies and products, baked beans and boiled, mashed and jacket potatoes and to be drinking coffee. In contrast children in the Northern region were least likely to be eating rice, coated chicken, raw and salad vegetables (not tomatoes or carrots). Children in Scotland were most likely to be eating chips, beef and beef products, canned fruit in syrup and drinking soft drinks and were least likely to be eating cheese, most types of vegetables and drinking fruit juice. *(Chapter 4)*

The differences in foods eaten were not reflected in differences in average daily energy intake since there were no significant differences in energy intake according to region. *(Chapter 5)*

There was almost no variation between children living in different regions in the proportion of energy they derived from protein, total carbohydrate and total fat. Only intakes of NSP and starch varied significantly by region, intakes of starch being lowest for children living in London and the South East and highest among those from the Central, South West and Wales region. Intakes of NSP were also highest for children in the Central, South West and Wales region, but were lowest among children in Scotland. There were very few differences in average intake of fatty acids between children living in different parts of Great Britain. Any differences were associated with the small differences in energy intake. *(Chapters 6 and 7)*

There were regional variations in the vitamin intakes of children. Children in Scotland had the lowest intakes of vitamin C and total carotene. Children in London and the South East together with children living in the Northern region of England had the lowest intakes of folate. In most cases these differences were still apparent after adjusting for any differences in energy intake. *(Chapter 8)*

Children living in London and the South East tended to have the highest intakes of minerals except that their intakes of sodium, chloride and iodine were on average among the lowest. In Scotland, the position was reversed. Even after adjusting for the small differences in energy intakes, the intakes of several minerals by children living in Scotland tended to be lower than in children living elsewhere. *(Chapter 9)*

There were no marked associations between the results for the blood haematology and region. However there were differences in the results from the water soluble vitamins measured in blood (apart from the EGRAC), with children from the Northern region having generally lower values than for children living elsewhere in Great Britain. *(Chapter 10)*

Boys living in Scotland and the Northern region of England had a BMI above the average but there was no significant difference in BMI for girls in the different regions. *(Chapter 11)*

Socio-economic characteristics

Children were classified according to the social class of head of household (based on their occupation), which for reporting was described as manual and non-manual backgrounds. Other measures of socio-economic status were based on the employment status of head of household, whether the household was receiving Family Credit and/or Income Support, and the mother's highest educational qualification level.

There were several differences in the consumption of foods between children from manual and non-manual backgrounds. Children from non-manual home backgrounds were more likely to have eaten rice, wholemeal bread, wholegrain and high-fibre breakfast cereals, and buns, cakes and pastries than were children from a manual home background although the average amounts eaten did not differ greatly. However children from a manual home background were more likely to have eaten white bread and non-wholegrain and high fibre breakfast cereals and in significantly greater amounts. There was a marked difference in consumption of fruit juice which was twice as likely in the non-manual group when compared with the manual group of children, while significantly more children from manual home backgrounds consumed tea. Children from non-manual homes were significantly more likely to be taking dietary supplements than children from manual homes. *(Chapter 4)*

Although there were differences in food consumption patterns, there were no significant differences in mean energy intake for children from manual and non-manual home backgrounds (manual 4830kJ/1148kcal, non-manual 4767kJ/1132kcal). Nor were there any significant differences related to the other indicators of socio-economic status. *(Chapter 5)*

Girls from a non-manual home background and with mothers with no formal educational qualifications tended to have a lower than average BMI but there was no significant difference between boys from different socio-economic backgrounds. *(Chapter 11)*

When carbohydrate intakes were related to indicators of socio-economic status, there was a significant trend for children from households of lower economic status to have lower average intakes of total sugars but higher starch intakes than other children. This relationship was consistent for measures based on mothers' educational qualifications, the employment status of the head of household, and social class. There was also a tendency for children from a manual social class background to have lower intakes of protein and higher absolute intakes of total fat and certain fatty acids (especially *cis* monounsaturated fatty acids). However the percentage energy from total fat was not significantly different for children from less economically advantaged backgrounds (with the exception of the group whose mothers had no formal educational qualifications where the contribution from fat was higher) than other children. *(Chapters 6 and 7)*

Lower intakes of most vitamins were recorded for children from manual home backgrounds. When the intakes were adjusted for differences between the groups in energy intake, the diets of children from manual backgrounds were found to have proportionately lower amounts of total carotene, niacin, vitamin B_{12}, vitamin C and E. Within the range of values recorded for blood levels of vitamins, there were associations with all vitamin status levels recorded (except the EGRAC) and socio-economic characteristics. Thus, except for the EGRAC, lowest values tended to be recorded in children from manual homes or where the head of household was not working, where parents were receiving Income Support and/or Family Credit or where the mother had a low level of educational qualifications. *(Chapters 8 and 10)*

Children from non-manual home backgrounds tended to have higher average intakes of most minerals except sodium and chloride for which higher average intakes were recorded in the diets of children from manual home backgrounds. Furthermore, children from manual home backgrounds had lower intakes than other children of many minerals even after adjusting for differences in energy intakes. *(Chapter 9)*

Most haematological analytes showed no variation by social class, employment status or receipt of benefits but there was an observed difference in mean levels of ferritin between samples from children whose head of household was working ($24\mu g/l$) and those from children where the head was economically inactive ($21\mu g/l$). *(Chapter 10)*

Family type

Children in the survey were ascribed to one of four family types for reporting purposes: married or cohabiting couple with one child; married or cohabiting couple with more than one child; lone parent with one child; lone parent with more than one child. Eighty two percent of the children were living with married or cohabiting adults (two-parent families) and only 18% were living with one parent (lone-parent families). A higher proportion of two-parent families had two or more children compared with lone-parent families, 73% compared with 60%. *(Chapter 3)*

There were no significant differences in mean energy intake according to family type, although the data suggest that intakes of children in lone-parent families tended to be higher than for children in two-parent families. Average daily energy intake for one child living in a two-parent family was 4680kJ (1112kcal), for a child that had siblings living in a two-parent family 4802kJ (1141kcal), for one child living in a lone-parent family 4959kJ (1181kcal) and for a child with siblings living in a one-parent family 4911kJ (1169kcal). The range of energy intakes for children in lone-parent families, particularly where there was only one child, was large; 2560kJ (610kcal) to 8341kJ (1986kcal) between the lower and upper 2.5 percentiles. *(Chapter 5)*

Differences in body weight, height and BMI between children from different family types were not statistically significant although single children (boys and girls) and girls with siblings in lone-parent families were slightly heavier than the average weight for all children and both boys and girls in two-parent families were slightly lighter. Children from lone-parent families were slightly taller than other children and single children (boys and girls) and girls with siblings in lone-parent families had slightly greater BMIs than the mean for all children. *(Chapter 11)*

Overall there was no significant variation in the average daily intake of carbohydrates and protein associated with family type nor did the proportion of energy derived from carbohydrates vary significantly. However children from lone-parent families where there was more than one child in the family had significantly higher intakes of starch than other children, but lower intakes of total sugars and non-milk extrinsic sugars (as compared with children from two-parent families with more than one child) *(Table 6.30)*. The mean daily intake of total sugars for children (single and with siblings) living in two-parent families was 88g, for one child living with one parent, 86g and for a child with siblings living with one parent, 81g. *(Chapter 6)*

There was a pattern of higher intakes of total fat and fatty acids by children in one-parent families compared with children in two-parent families, and a general tendency for children with siblings to have somewhat higher intakes than children with no siblings. Some differences in the percentage of energy derived from total fat and fatty acids between the groups were evident but they were small. For example, the mean percentage of food energy derived from total fat for one child in a two-parent family was 35.9%, for a child with siblings in a two-parent family 35.8%, for a single child in a one-parent family 36.1% and for a child with siblings in a one-parent family 36.5% *(Table 7.28)*.   *(Chapter 7)*

Children in one-parent families with more than one child had the lowest absolute intakes of both total carotene and vitamin C. After adjusting for variation in energy intakes vitamin C levels for these children were still lower than for other children. Children who had brothers or sisters, both in one-parent and two-parent families, had lower intakes of most vitamins than other children *(Table 8.52)*.   *(Chapter 8)*

Average intake of most minerals varied little according to family type. However there was a tendency for absolute intakes of calcium, phosphorus and potassium to be lower and intakes of sodium and chloride to be higher in children from one-parent families with brothers and sisters than those of other children. Those differences remained even after allowing for differences in energy intake.   *(Chapter 9)*

There were no clear associations between mean levels of the haematological analytes and family type, nor with whether the child was an only child, or had siblings. Levels of water soluble vitamins assayed (except the EGRAC) were generally lower for children from one-parent families compared with those for other children. The variation was not generally as marked as for the other socio-economic characteristics, but levels of vitamin C showed the largest relative differences, for example comparing two-parent families with one child and lone-parent families with more than one child the vitamin C levels for the children in the survey were 75.2μmol/l and 58.4μmol/l respectively.   *(Chapter 10)*

References

1 Gregory J, Foster K, Tyler H, Wiseman M. *The Dietary and Nutritional Survey of British Adults*. HMSO (London, 1990).

2 Department of Health and Social Security. Report on Health and Social Subjects: 10. *A Nutrition Survey of Pre-school Children 1967–68*. HMSO (London, 1975).

3 Thomas M, Goddard E, Hickman M, and Hunter P. *1992 General Household Survey*. HMSO (London, 1994).

4 Population Estimates Unit, OPCS, Crown Copyright (unpublished data). In mid-1992 the number of children born in 1988, 1989, 1990 and 1991 and living in Great Britain was estimated to be 3,019,644. Of these children 25% were born in each of the four years showing an equal distribution in the population from which the survey sample was drawn.

5 Hinds K, Gregory J. *The National Diet and Nutrition Survey: Children aged 1½ to 4½ years. Volume 2. Report of the Dental Survey*. HMSO (London, 1995).

6 Department of Health. Report on Health and Social Subjects: 41. *Dietary Reference Values for Food Energy and Nutrients for the United Kingdom*. HMSO (London, 1991).

7 White A, Davies PSW. *Feasibility Study for the National Diet and Nutrition Survey of Children aged 1½ to 4½ years*. OPCS (1994) (NM22).

8 Department of Health and Social Security. Report on Health and Social Subjects: 15. *Recommended Daily Amounts of Food Energy and Nutrients for Groups of People in the United Kingdom*. HMSO (London, 1979).

9 World Health Organisation. WHO Technical Report Series No: 503 *Nutritional Anaemias*. WHO (Geneva, 1972).

List of tables and figures

page

Chapter 2 Response rates and characteristics of respondents

2.1	Response to the household sifts to identify children eligible for the dietary survey	5
2.2	Response to the dental survey in relation to response to the dietary survey	6
2.3	Response to different components of the dental survey	6
2.4	Response to different components of the dental examination	6
2.5	Response to different components of the dental survey by sex and age	7
2.6	Age distribution of children with dental interviews and dental interviews and full examinations, by sex compared with the dietary survey interview sample	7
2.7	Social class distribution of children with dental interviews, dental interviews and full examinations and dietary interviews, compared with sub-sample from the 1992 GHS	8
2.8	Regional distribution of children in the dental sample compared with the general population	8
2.9	Social class distribution by region; dental sample and sub-sample from 1992 GHS compared	9
2.10	Highest educational qualification of children's mothers by age of child	9
2.11	Highest educational qualification of children's mothers by social class of head of household and age of child	9
2.12	Family type by age of child	9
2.13	Whether mother worked and who looked after child, by age of child	10
2.14	Employment status of head of household by age of child	10
2.15	Whether parents in receipt of Income Support or Family Credit, by age of child	10

Chapter 3 Condition of young children's teeth

3.1	Proportion of children with any active decay, filled teeth, teeth missing due to decay and any decay experience, by age	11
3.2	Proportion of children with any active decay, filled teeth, teeth missing due to decay and any decay experience, by age and social class of head of household	12
3.3	Proportion of children with any active decay, filled teeth, teeth missing due to decay and any decay experience, by age and region	12
3.4	Proportion of children in Wales with any active decay, filled teeth, teeth missing due to decay and any decay experience, by age	12
3.5	Proportion of children in England with any active decay, filled teeth, teeth missing due to decay and any decay experience, by age	13
3.6	Proportion of children with any active decay, filled teeth, teeth missing due to decay and any decay experience, by age and mother's highest educational qualification	13
3.7	Proportion of children with any active decay, filled teeth, teeth missing due to decay and any decay experience, by age and family type	13
3.8	Proportion of children with any active decay, filled teeth, teeth missing due to decay and any decay experience, by age and employment status of head of household	13
3.9	Proportion of children with any active decay, filled teeth, teeth missing due to decay and any decay experience, by age and whether parents in receipt of Income Support or Family Credit	14
3.10	Proportion of children with any active decay, filled teeth, teeth missing due to decay and any decay experience, by age and social class of head of household and whether parents in receipt of Income Support or Family Credit	14
3.11	Proportion of children with any decay experience by age and the child's position in the family, whether mother did any paid work in the last week and whether child attending a nursery school or playgroup	15
3.12	Proportion of children with decay into the dental pulp by age and social class of head of household, region, mother's highest educational qualification, family type, employment status of head of household and whether parents in receipt of Income Support or Family Credit	15
3.13	The mean number of teeth with any active decay, evidence of treatment (filled or missing teeth) and any decay experience by age	16
3.14	The mean number of teeth with any decay experience by age and social class of head of household, region, mother's highest educational qualification, family type, employment status of head of household and whether parents in receipt of Income Support or Family Credit	16

3.15   The mean number of teeth with any decay experience, for children aged $3^1/_2$ to $4^1/_2$ years with
        some decay experience by age and social class of head of household, region, mother's highest
        educational qualification, family type, employment status of head of household and whether parents
        in receipt of Income Support or Family Credit   17
3.16   The number of teeth with decay experience by age   17
3.17   The mean number of teeth with decay into the dental pulp by age, for all children, those with any
        decay and those with any decay into the dental pulp   17
3.18   Proportion of children with any active decay and decay experience on molars, incisors and canines,
        by age   18
3.19   Proportion of children with any decay experience on molars, incisors and canines for children aged
        $3^1/_2$ to $4^1/_2$ years with some decay experience by age and social class of head of household, region,
        mother's highest educational qualification, family type, employment status of head of household
        and whether parents in receipt of Income Support or Family Credit   18
3.20   Proportion of dental decay which was treated and untreated among children in the survey, by age 18
3.21   Proportion of dental decay which was treated among children of different ages, by social class of head of
        household, region, mother's highest educational qualification, family type, employment status of head of
        household and whether parents in receipt of Income Support or Family Credit   19

Chapter 4 Dental care and advice

4.1   Visits to the dentist by age of child   21
4.2   Visits to the dentist by social class of head of household and age of child   21
4.3   Visits to the dentist by region and age of child   21
4.4   Visits to the dentist by mother's highest educational qualification and age of child   22
4.5   Advice on dental care received by parents, by age of child   22
4.6   Advice on dental care received by parents by social class of head of household and age of child   22
4.7   Advice on dental care received by parents, by region and age of child   22
4.8   Sources of advice for parents who received advice on aspects of dental care, by age of child   23
4.9   Teething difficulties by sex and age of child   23
4.10   Type of teething aids used by age of child   23
4.11   Teething difficulties and type of teething aids used by age of child   24
4.12   Proportion of children who used different teething aids by social class of head of household and
        age of child   24
4.13   Type of teething aids used by mother's highest educational qualification and age of child   24
4.14   Whether toothbrushing started by age of child   24
4.15   Age when toothbrushing started by age of child   25
4.16   Age when toothbrushing started by social class of head of household and age of child   25
4.17   Who brushes child's teeth by sex and age of child   25
4.18   Who brushes child's teeth by social class of head of household and age of child   25
4.19   Who cleans child's teeth by mother's highest educational qualification and age of child   25
4.20   Frequency of toothbrushing by sex and age of child   26
4.21   Frequency of toothbrushing by social class of head of household and age of child   26
4.22   Times of day when teeth brushed by age of child   26
4.23   Times of day when teeth brushed by frequency of brushing and age of child   26
4.24   Fluoride concentration of toothpaste used, by age of child   27
4.25   Fluoride concentration of toothpaste used, by social class of head of household and age of child 27
4.26   Fluoride concentration of toothpaste used, by mother's highest educational qualification and age of child   27
4.27   Fluoride concentration of toothpaste used, by region and age of child   28
4.28   Size of toothbrush used by age of child   28
4.29   Amount of toothpaste used by age of child   28
4.30   Fluoride concentration of toothpaste and amount used by age of child   28
4.31   Fluoride concentration of toothpaste and amount used by social class of head of household   29
4.32   Use of fluoride supplements by age of child   29
4.33   Use of fluoride supplements by social class of head of household and age of child   29
4.34   Use of fluoride supplements by region and age of child   29
4.35   Age when child started using fluoride supplements by age of child   29
4.36   Use of fluoride supplements by whether parents received advice to give child fluoride and age of child   30
4.37   Mother's dental attendance pattern by age of child   30
4.38   Child's visits to the dentist by mother's dental attendance pattern and age of child   30

**Chapter 5 The use of bottles, dinky feeders and dummies and the consumption of foods and drinks
             containing sugars**

5.1   Whether children had ever used, or currently used bottles, by age   31
5.2   Whether children had ever used, or currently used bottles, by age and social class of head of household   31
5.3   Age when bottle users started and stopped use by age   31
5.4   Whether children currently used bottles during the day and the frequency of use, by age   32
5.5   Whether children currently used bottles at night and the frequency of use, by age   32
5.6   Usual drinks consumed from bottles during the night, among children using bottles at night at the time of
        interview, by age   32
5.7   Whether children had ever used, or currently used dinky feeders, by age   32
5.8   Age when dinky feeder users started and stopped use by age   32
5.9   Drinks which children who were using dinky feeders at the time of interview, or who had used them in the
        past, were reported to consume from them most frequently during the day   33
5.10   Whether children had ever used, or currently used dummies, by age   33
5.11   Age when dummy users started and stopped use by age   33
5.12   Whether children were reported to have a drink in bed at the time of interview and the frequency of
        having drinks in bed, by age   34
5.13   How often children were reported to have a drink in bed at the time of interview, and the usual drinks
        taken to bed, by age   34
5.14   How often children were reported to have a drink in bed at the time of interview, and the drinking
        vessels they usually used, by age   34
5.15   Drinks children were reported to consume from different vessels most often in bed at the time of
        interview, by age   34
5.16   Whether children were reported to have a drink in bed at the time of interview and the frequency of
        having drinks in bed, by social class of head of household and age   34
5.17   Types of drink consumed in bed or during the night among children who had drinks in bed, by social
        class of head of household and age   35
5.18   Whether children were reported to have food in bed at the time of interview and the frequency with
        which they had food at night, by age   35
5.19   Types of food consumed in bed or during the night, by age   35
5.20   Frequency with which children aged $1^1/_2$ to $2^1/_2$ years were reported to consume various foods
        containing sugars   36
5.21   Frequency with which children aged $2^1/_2$ to $3^1/_2$ years were reported to consume various foods
        containing sugars   36
5.22   Frequency with which children aged $3^1/_2$ to $4^1/_2$ years were reported to consume various foods
        containing sugars   36
5.23   Proportion of children who were reported to consume sugar confectionery and carbonated
        drinks on at least most days of the week, by social class of head of household and age   37
5.24   Average daily frequency of consumption of selected foods containing sugars and average daily intake
        of these foods and selected nutrients, by age   37
5.25   Upper and lower percentiles for the frequency of consumption of selected foods containing sugars and
        the average daily intake of these foods and selected nutrients, by age   38
5.26   Average weekly household expenditure on chocolates and sweets, by age   39
5.27   Average weekly household expenditure on chocolates and sweets, by social class of head of household
        and age of child   39

Chapter 6 Variations in patterns of decay
6.1   Proportion of children with any active decay, filled teeth, teeth missing due to decay and any decay
        experience, by age and age when started toothbrushing   41
6.2   Proportion of children with any active decay, filled teeth, teeth missing due to decay and any decay
        experience, by age and frequency of toothbrushing   41
6.3   Proportion of children with any active decay, filled teeth, teeth missing due to decay and any decay
        experience, by age and who brushes child's teeth   42
6.4   Proportion of children with any active decay, filled teeth, teeth missing due to decay and any decay
        experience, by age and child's experience of visiting the dentist   42
6.5   Proportion of children with experience of decay according to whether advice on dental care received
        by parents, by age of child   42
6.6   Proportion of children with any active decay, filled teeth, teeth missing due to decay and any decay
        experience, by age and use of fluoride supplements   43
6.7   Proportion of children with any active decay, filled teeth, teeth missing due to decay and any decay
        experience, by age and age started using fluoride supplements   43

6.8   Proportion of children with any active decay, filled teeth, teeth missing due to decay and any decay
        experience, by age and mother's dental attendance pattern   43
6.9   Proportion of children with any decay experience by age and whether used a bottle, dinky feeder,
        or dummy   44
6.10   Proportion of children with any decay experience by age and night-time drinking practices at the time
        of interview   45
6.11   Proportion of children with any active decay, filled teeth, teeth missing due to decay and any decay
        experience, by age and average weekly household expenditure on chocolates and sweets   45
6.12   Proportion of children with experience of decay by age and the frequency with which they were reported
        to consume various foods containing sugars   46
6.13   Proportion of children with experience of decay by age and the frequency with which they were reported
        to consume various drinks containing sugars   47
6.14   Average daily frequency of consumption of selected foods containing sugars, and average daily intake of
        these foods and selected nutrients, for children with and without experience of caries; children aged
        $2\frac{1}{2}$ to $3\frac{1}{2}$ years   47
6.15   Average daily frequency of consumption of selected foods containing sugars, and average daily
        intake of these foods and selected nutrients, for children with and without experience of caries;
        children aged $3\frac{1}{2}$ to $4\frac{1}{2}$ years   48
6.16   Proportion of children with any decay experience for children whose average daily frequency of
        consumption and intakes of selected foods and nutrients, were below the 10th percentile and above
        the 90th percentile value, by age   48
6.17   Background, dental care and dietary behaviour variables found to be independently related to decay
        experience, by age   49
6.18   Variables found to be independently related to decay experience, by age   50
6.19   The proportion of children with decay experience according to the frequency with which children were
        reported to consume sugar confectionery and carbonated drinks, and the frequency of toothbrushing,
        by age   50

Chapter 7 Trauma to the incisors and erosion of the upper incisors
7.1   Proportion of children with experience of trauma to the incisors, by sex and age   52
7.2   Proportion of children with experience of trauma to the incisors in the upper and lower jaws by age 52
7.3   The mean number of incisors with experience of trauma for all children and children with some trauma,
        by age   52
7.4   Types of trauma recorded for children with some trauma to the incisors, by age   52
7.5   Proportion of children with any erosion recorded on buccal and palatal surfaces of incisors and with
        any erosion into dentine or pulp, by age   53
7.6   The mean number of teeth with any erosion and erosion into dentine or pulp for buccal and palatal
        surfaces; means shown for all children and for children with some erosion of type specified, by age 53
7.7   Proportion of children with erosion on individual deciduous teeth by age   54
7.8   Area of the tooth surface affected by erosion on eroded teeth   54

Appendix C Tables associated with Chapter 5: data on past use of bottles
1   Use of bottles at night immediately prior to stopping use by children no longer using bottles at the
        time of interview   111
2   Use of bottles in the day immediately prior to stopping use by children no longer using bottles at the
        time of interview   111
3   Drinks usually consumed from bottles at night immediately prior to stopping use, by children who had
        used bottles at night but were no longer doing so at the time of interview   111
4   Drinks usually consumed from bottles during the day immediately prior to stopping use, by children who
        had used bottles during the day but were no longer doing so at the time of interview   111

**Appendix D Tables associated with Chapter 6: The mean number of teeth with experience of decay
              in relation to various dental care and dietary behaviour variables**
1   The mean number of teeth with any decay experience by age and age started toothbrushing, frequency
        of toothbrushing and who brushes child's teeth   112
2   The mean number of teeth with any decay experience by age and child's visits to the dentist and advice
        received about dental care   112
3   The mean number of teeth with any decay experience by age and whether child given fluoride
        supplements, age started using fluoride supplements, mother's dental attendance pattern and average
        weekly household expenditure on sweets and chocolates   113
4   The mean number of teeth with any decay experience by age and whether child ever used a bottle,
        dinky feeder or dummy   113

5   The mean number of teeth with any decay experience by age and night-time drinking practices at
     the time of interview   113
6   The mean number of teeth with experience of decay by age and the frequency with which children
     were reported to consume sugar confectionery, chocolate confectionery, biscuits, cakes and ice cream
     or ice lollies (from the dietary interview)   114
7   The mean number of teeth with experience of decay by age and the frequency with which children were
     reportedto consume carbonated drinks, blackcurrant drinks and fruit juice (from the dietary interview),   114
8   The mean number of teeth with any decay experience according to the frequency of consumption of
     selected foods containing sugars and the average daily intake of these foods and selected nutrients,
     by age of child; data presented for those with intakes below the 10th percentile value and above the
     90th percentile value   114

**Appendix E Tables associated with Chapter 7: The proportion of children with erosion in relation to various
             background and behavioral characteristics**
1   Proportion of children with erosion, by age and social class of the head of household   115
2   Proportion of children with erosion, by age and mother's highest educational qualification   115
3   Proportion of children with erosion, by age and whether parents in receipt of Income Support or
     Family Credit   115
4   Proportion of children with erosion, by age and region   116
5   Proportion of children with erosion, by age and age when started toothbrushing   116
6   Proportion of children with erosion, by age and frequency of toothbrushing   116
7   Proportion of children with erosion, by age and who brushes child's teeth   117
8   Proportion of children with erosion, by age and whether ever used fluoride supplements   117
9   Proportion of children with erosion, by age and whether ever used a bottle   117
10   Proportion of children with erosion, by age and whether ever used a dinky feeder   117
11   Proportion of children with erosion, by age and whether ever used a dummy   118
12   Proportion of children with erosion, by age and average weekly household spending on chocolates
     and sweets   118
13   Proportion of children with erosion, by age and frequency of consuming sugar confectionery   118
14   Proportion of children with erosion, by age and frequency of consuming carbonated drinks   118
15   Proportion of children with erosion, by age and frequency of having a drink in bed
     (at the time of interview)   119
16   Proportion of children with erosion, by age and vessel used when having a drink in bed   119
17   Proportion of children with erosion, by age and drink usually had when drinking in bed   119
18   Proportion of children with any buccal erosion into dentine or pulp for children whose average daily
     frequency of consumption and intakes of certain foods and nutrients, were below the 10th percentile
     value and above the 90th percentile value, by age   120
19   Proportion of children with any palatal erosion into dentine or pulp for children whose average daily
     frequency of consumption and intakes of certain foods and nutrients, were below the 10th percentile
     value and above the 90th percentile value, by age   120

Appendix F Sampling errors
1   True standard errors and design factors for socio-demographic characteristics of the dental sample   122
2   Proportion of children with different dental conditions and the associated standard errors and
     design factors   123
3   Proportion of children with different patterns of toothbrushing and the associated standard errors and
     design factors   124
4   True standard errors and design factors for certain behavioral characteristics of the dental sample
5   Standard errors and design factors associated with different frequencies of having a drink in bed at
     night and the type of vessel used for night-time drink   125
6   Standard errors and design factors associated with having different drinks in bed at night   125
7   Average daily intake of selected foods containing sugars and certain nutrients and the associated
     standard errors and design factors   126
8   Average daily frequency of consumption of selected foods containing sugars and the associated
     standard errors and design factors   127

List of figures

Chapter 3 Condition of young children's teeth
3.1   The distribution of tooth condition around the mouth, by age   20

Appendix G
G1   Standard Regions of England, Scotland, and Wales, and aggregated regions for analysis   131